The Science of Movement, Exercise, and Mental Health

by the same author

Body Mind Movement
An Evidence-Based Approach to Mindful Movement
Jennifer Pilotti
Forewords by Joanne Elphinston, Christine Ruffolo, and Kathryn Bruni-Young
ISBN 978 1 91208 589 7
eISBN 978 1 91208 590 3

of related interest

Yoga for Mental Health
Edited by Heather Mason and Kelly Birch
Forewords by B N Gangadhar and Timothy McCall
ISBN 978 1 90914 135 3
eISBN 978 1 91208 526 2

THE SCIENCE of MOVEMENT, EXERCISE, and MENTAL HEALTH

Jennifer Pilotti

Illustrated by Sevinc Gurmen

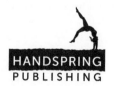

HANDSPRING
PUBLISHING

First published in Great Britain in 2023 by Handspring
Publishing, an imprint of Jessica Kingsley Publishers
Part of John Murray Press

2

*Disclaimer: The information contained in this book is not intended to replace the services of
trained medical professionals or to be a substitute for medical advice. The complementary therapy
described in this book may not be suitable for everyone to follow. You are advised to consult a
doctor before embarking on any complementary therapy programme and on any matters relating
to your health, and in particular on any matters that may require diagnosis or medical attention.*

A CIP catalogue record for this title is available from the
British Library and the Library of Congress

ISBN 978 1 83997 773 2
eISBN 978 1 83997 774 9

Printed and bound in Great Britain by CPI Group, Croydon CR0 4YY

Jessica Kingsley Publishers' policy is to use papers that are natural, renewable
and recyclable products and made from wood grown in sustainable
forests. The logging and manufacturing processes are expected to conform
to the environmental regulations of the country of origin.

Handspring Publishing
Carmelite House
50 Victoria Embankment
London EC4Y 0DZ

www.handspringpublishing.com

John Murray Press
Part of Hodder & Stoughton Limited
An Hachette UK Company

Contents

Introduction

Anxiety is an emotion, a feeling of worry, a sense of tense muscles for no particular reason. It's a shortness of breath, a rapid heart rate, and the nagging sense that something is wrong. It manifests in a variety of ways. Maybe your stomach is upset for no obvious reason, or the nagging pain in your low back never leaves, or you just accept that your tight neck is chronic and you are never going to be able to take a deep breath again.

Feelings of anxiety once in a while are normal. As humans, worrying and forecasting "what if" is part of how we evolved to survive. However, when feelings and thoughts associated with anxiety become habitual, they can have a profound impact on physical health and well-being, affecting digestion, muscular tension, heart rate, and breathing patterns. Without any form of intervention, anxiety also affects the rest of our lives, including the things we need to thrive, like relationships with other people and the ability to exercise in a way that feels safe.

There are other emotions that affect physical well-being. Depression, for instance, is heavy, like a weighted vest that engulfs you, dragging you down into a hyperbolic abyss. It's hard to remove and its memory is even more difficult to shake once it's gone, as though at any point it could reattach itself firmly to your body and never leave.

This is a book about exercise and mental health, specifically how exercise impacts mental health. There are physical conditions that predispose people to anxiety and depression; anxiety and depression can also predispose people to certain physical conditions. Learning how to

7

build stamina, strength, and balance in a progressive way is like placing the right key into a lock and having it fit. Unlocking the metaphorical door through the appropriate exercise intervention can change not only your relationship with your physical self, but also how you respond to and interact with the environment around you. As you begin to feel more secure in your physical abilities and more confident in your ability to navigate the physical world, you feel a sense of strength and resilience that permeates your emotional self. The mind and the body are not separate; changing the body, then, changes the mind.

For ease of reading, the book is split into two sections. Part I reviews the why: what does research on exercise and mental health show and what are the potential mechanisms for why it works?

Part II explores how to apply the concepts while exploring different exercise modalities and their relationship to mental health and well-being. You will find sample programs, ideas for exercise progressions, and ways to help people become comfortable with exploring movement.

I have been working with clients in a one-on-one setting for over 20 years. During that time, I have worked with a number of clients who have experienced chronic anxiety, depression, and/or post-traumatic stress. Witnessing the long-term effects of a thoughtful exercise program has been incredibly rewarding and has spurred me on to spend countless hours reading research and essays, talking to people, and applying concepts in my own practice. There is no one-size-fits-all approach, but I hope the ideas and progressions outlined on these pages will help you see movement as necessary for more than physical well-being.

PART I

THE SCIENCE

CHAPTER 1

The Science and Concepts

If you work as a mental health care professional, much of the science will not be new to you; however, it's helpful to be reminded of how the nervous system works and how it is impacted by anxiety, depression, and trauma. The information about the impact of movement on mental health will reinforce these connections.

> My ten-year-old sister, circa 1991: "I think I have AIDS."
> Twelve-year-old me: "You don't have AIDS."
> Sister, concerned: "How do you know? I have a bump on the back of my neck. That could be from AIDS and I could be dying."

Twelve years later...

> Thirty-five-year-old client: "I think I have diabetes."
> Me, surprised: "Why do you think that?"
> Client: "Because I've been drinking lots of water lately."
> Me: "Do you think maybe you're just thirsty because you've been exercising more?"

Anxiety is an emotional state that is non-discriminatory; it affects people of all ages. It can appear as an upset stomach before doing something uncomfortable, or a chronic feeling of unease, breathlessness, or elevated heart rate that is intimately linked to a sense of worry and fear.

It's estimated that one in three children and adolescents will experience anxiety-related symptoms before they turn 18 (Cohodes & Gee, 2017). Five years after my sister was convinced she had AIDS, she ended up with shingles. The doctors missed it initially because nobody that young gets shingles. The anxiety she regularly experienced had taken a toll on her immune system.

If you live in the United States, there is a 33 percent chance you will have an anxiety disorder during your lifetime. The client above used to walk around with anti-anxiety medications in her purse just in case she felt a panic attack coming on. Anxiety disorders are often chronic and are a leading source of disability worldwide (Knight & Depue, 2019).

Anxiety is different than fear, because fear is a phasic response to an immediate and identifiable stressor. Anxiety, on the other hand, is a prolonged state of apprehension caused by an uncertain or prospective threat. Have you ever watched as something potentially injurious is about to happen, like a car crash or mugging? That activates your fear response. Have you ever found yourself lying awake at night, imagining a potentially emotional situation like your divorced parents coming to your wedding and having a huge fight, your child not getting into college, or your house burning down? That is anxiety. These scenarios may or may not happen, but they leave you with a feeling of dread.

My sister is prone to thinking something catastrophic might happen. What keeps these thoughts from keeping her up at night? Riding a Peloton bike or participating in her boot camp class.

The client I mentioned above used to have very real panic attacks at weddings and on planes. Her symptoms gradually decreased as she incorporated more and more movement into her life, until she no longer feared she would have a panic attack in a public place or had to run to the bathroom to remove clothing so she could breathe.

A Brief Review of the Nervous System

In order to fully understand how movement and anxiety are linked, it helps to review the physiology of the nervous system, which regulates our actions and behaviors. The nervous system is the collection of nerve and brain cells, or neurons, that converse with each other, sharing information in the form of hormones and synapses between cells. This results in feelings and behavior. Behavior can be thought of as a series of actions that are taken to achieve a specific goal. All behavior requires some form of movement, so the body plays an integral role in the actions we perform to navigate the world around us.

The nervous system is divided into two main parts. The central nervous system (CNS) is the brain and the spinal cord. The peripheral nervous system (PNS) is everything else, including the somatic nervous system (SoNS) and the autonomic nervous system (ANS).

The brain and the spinal cord are where conscious thought occurs, patterns are recognized, and all of the afferent, or sensory, input from the PNS is assessed and the appropriate action (or behavior) is determined based on the input received. The PNS then signals the appropriate action, and motor neurons are excited, causing movement.

Another way to think of this is: information comes in, the CNS figures out what to do with that information, and the appropriate action or behavior occurs.

The part of the PNS that receives all of the information about the environment is called the sensory, or afferent, branch of the nervous system. The part of the nervous system that tells which muscles to move is the motor, or efferent, branch of the nervous system. When I was first learning the branches of the nervous system, I used the acronym SAME: sensory/afferent, motor/efferent.

You are taking in senses from lots of different places all of the time. Your eyes, nose, skin, ears, tongue, muscles, heart, and digestive system are constantly sending information that influences how you feel, think, and move.

The sensory part of the SoNS is made up of specialized nerves that pick up information about pressure, temperature, and pain. They are information gatherers, submitting all information to the CNS so motor neurons can be triggered, causing movement (Cuevas, 2007). The afferent receptors are the input; the efferent receptors are the output.

The PNS also consists of the ANS, which has two branches: the sympathetic nervous system (SNS) and the parasympathetic nervous system (PSNS). The ANS controls the heart, blood vessels, glands, organs, and smooth muscle (smooth muscle is muscle that is found in viscera, while skeletal muscle is muscle that is found on the skeleton). There are still afferent and efferent fibers, so input is received from the viscera, which triggers the signal to manage smooth muscle and vascular tone. The ANS and the SoNS are intertwined; if you go from standing to sprinting, the SoNS is what allows the muscles in the legs and arms to begin moving rapidly in a coordinated fashion, while the ANS sends information to the heart to beat faster and tells the blood vessels to dilate, allowing the blood (which carries oxygen) to move more quickly to the working muscles (Cuevas, 2011).

There is no separation between the components of the PNS and the CNS. What happens in the PNS affects what happens in the CNS and vice versa. This connection between the mind and the body implies that altering what's happening in the body will impact what's happening in the brain.

This suggests that you can alter your emotional experience through doing something physical. As you will see in later chapters, your physical choices can create a cascade of emotional changes.

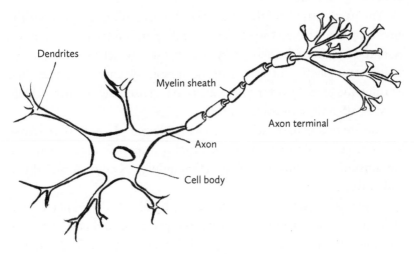

NERVE CELL

Nerves are the physical housing of the bundle of fibers that transmit information using either electrical or chemical signals. If you were to look at a cadaver and identify a nerve, you would discover a long, wiry-looking object that branches off into different areas of the body. Along the outside of the nerve axon, or fiber, is an electrical insulator called myelin. These myelin sheaths allow neurons to conduct impulses from one to another in a continuous fashion that requires very little energy, creating effective communication between the different systems of the body (Morell & Quarles, 1999).

When the myelin sheath is damaged, communication between the nerve cells slows down. Though it is possible for new myelin to cover the axon, in a process called remyelination, these sheaths are generally thinner and shorter than the myelin that is generated during our development. In diseases like multiple sclerosis, remyelination fails, and the axon remains uncovered, vulnerable to degeneration. This results in a number of neurological symptoms, including visual loss, cognitive dysfunction, motor weakness, and pain (Susuki, 2010).

The nerves that comprise the PNS mostly originate from the spinal cord, the part of the CNS that is a continuation of the brainstem and extends the length of the spinal column. It is protected by the body structures of the vertebral column and is covered with three membranes (Nogradi & Vrbova, 2000–2013). Nerves exit the spinal cord via an opening in the vertebrae called the intervertebral foramina (along with arteries, veins, and ligaments), and each nerve has two nerve roots: sensory and motor. The sensory nerve root is ascending because it carries information up to the brainstem and brain, while the motor nerve root is descending, carrying information away from the brainstem and brain to the periphery.

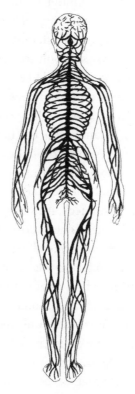

PERIPHERAL NERVOUS SYSTEM

Let's say you wanted to open the door of the refrigerator to assess its contents before making your grocery list. Let's assume you are standing facing the refrigerator door. The sensory information from the floor, your eyes, and the cells in your joints and muscles that sense joint position is all sent up the spinal cord to the brain. Based on this information, the brain determines the appropriate joint sequence needed to open the door and how much force is required. This information is sent down the spinal cord and out to the muscles, and movement happens. This happens so quickly you don't have time to consider whether you want to open the refrigerator a different way, because the behavior of opening the refrigerator has been practiced so often it feels automatic.

Cranial nerves are also part of the PNS, with the exception of the optic nerve, which isn't a true nerve but an extension of the brain tract (Snyder *et al.*, 2018). The optic nerve is therefore a direct extension of the brain, directly enervating the eye. It is responsible for vision (Rea, 2014; Barral & Croibier, 2009). Vision works with the vestibular system to keep you upright. You can begin to feel this relationship by placing your fingers at the base of the skull, right at the place where it's about to meet the spine. Move your eyes in different directions while keeping your head still (check in to make sure you aren't clenching your jaw and you are continuing to breathe). You will likely feel movement beneath your fingers as you move your eyes. Your neck muscles are responding to the change in eye position, ensuring that your head is stable as your eyes move. We will discuss balance more in Chapter 4 when we discuss enriched environments. Interestingly, the optic nerve is purely a sensory nerve (cranial nerve III is responsible for motor control of the eye).

There are 12 pairs of cranial nerves. They control motor and sensory functions of the head and neck, including smell, balance, sound, speech, the tongue, and, as mentioned above, the eye (Romano *et al.*, 2019). The optic nerve isn't the only cranial nerve that just relays sensory information to the brain; the olfactory nerve and the vestibulocochlear nerve, which provide information about smell and sound/balance, respectively, don't have a motor branch. Some of the cranial nerves have solely efferent branches, responsible for only motor output. Others are like the spinal nerves and are mixed use, with both afferent and efferent branches (Sonne & Lopez-Ojeda, 2019).

One of the cranial nerves that has both afferent and efferent functions is cranial nerve XI, aka the accessory spinal nerve. It activates the intrinsic laryngeal muscle fibers, which causes vocal cord movement. It also contracts the sternocleidomastoid and trapezius muscles and provides sensory information about these areas (Bordoni *et al.*, 2020). The accessory spinal nerve exits the spinal cord at the jugular foramen at the first cervical vertebrae (C1) with cranial nerve X, the vagus nerve (Felton *et al.*, 2016).

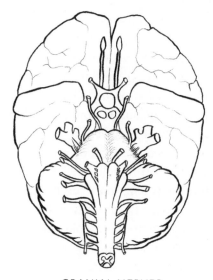

CRANIAL NERVES

TRY THIS: Tighten the back of your throat and then relax it. Motor output from your accessory spinal nerve gives you the ability to do this. Now shrug your shoulders a few times. This movement is also controlled by the accessory spinal nerve. Finally, tilt your right ear towards your right shoulder and turn your nose towards your right shoulder. This, too, is controlled by the accessory spinal nerve. These are three seemingly different movements that all originate neurologically from the same place.

The vagus nerve is the longest cranial nerve in the body (Kenny & Bordoni, 2019). It has sensory and motor branches and has a variety of functions, including transmitting sensory information from the heart, lungs, and upper gastrointestinal tract. It also carries parasympathetic fibers to the heart, upper respiratory tract, and gastrointestinal tract, which means it's activated when you are relaxed or your PSNS is activated.

Its name comes from the Latin word *vagor*, which means wandering (Rea, 2014).

Reflex versus Learned Behavior

When an action happens unconsciously, in a predictable way, this is generally thought of as a reflex. Researchers characterize reflexes as consistently performed subconscious reactions to external stimuli. When a doctor hits your knee with a hammer, for instance, the leg kick that occurs is a consistent, repeatable response to the sudden tap of the hammer (Fischer & Truog, 2015). This differs from asking someone to kick their leg, an action that is learned and will mean many different things to different people depending on their athletic backgrounds. Asking someone to kick their leg will also result in variation between repetitions, even in professional soccer players or football kickers.

Learned behavior differs from reflexive behavior in that it happens consciously, even though it sometimes feels like the behaviors we have learned are automatic. Asking the professional soccer player to kick his leg will result in a fast response that looks smooth and coordinated. That's because the behavior has been practiced so often it's automatic. The neurons have fired together so many times that they communicate rapidly, with minor deviations each time. If you ask someone who rarely performs kicking motions to kick their leg, the action will occur more slowly, with larger deviation between each repetition because the neurons that perform the action aren't used to conversing with each other. But with practice, the neurons will begin to grow accustomed to communicating, sending faster impulses as the pathways between each other become more worn, like a well-trodden trail.

This inherent plasticity of the nervous system means learning can occur across the lifespan and, while we can't change the knee-jerk response to the hammer, we can change conscious behavior, as well as behavior that is seemingly unconscious but is actually just a deeply ingrained habit, something that is so entrenched we don't feel the movement when it occurs. Learning to feel a habituated motor response when specific situations occur is the first step to being able to change the response.

Conveniently, the nervous system is the foundation for everything we do, so if neurons can continue to learn to communicate rapidly across the course of our lives, allowing us to learn new skills and adopt new behaviors, the benefits will be multi-faceted. The entire physiological system will be impacted, from the heart rate and how we breathe, to how our muscles contract and disperse load across the skeleton, to our learned responses to specific situations. We are capable of learning to recognize these internal patterns and choosing whether our learned response is serving us in the current moment. The ability to learn is, perhaps, one of the greatest tools we have for combatting the stresses of everyday life.

Top-Down versus Bottom-Up Processing

How you respond to the world and the sensory information you are receiving is complex. You can analyze the information and make a decision about how to respond consciously. You can also respond intuitively, allowing the sensory information you receive from the internal and external environments to inform your behavior and movements. These two types of processing are called top-down and bottom-up, respectively.

What actually happens is a combination of the two, since the different areas of the brain responsible for processing the environment work together (Rauss & Pourtois, 2013). Have you ever sniffed the leftover casserole in the fridge and intuitively turned away without thinking about it, only realizing a moment later that the food smelt bad? Or have you ever walked to the coffee shop on your lunch break and, for reasons that were inexplicable to you at the time, realized that all you wanted was white bread—definitely not latte—and then, 12 hours later, realized that you had the flu? These are examples of processing that occurs mostly from the bottom up. Your reaction and behavior is based on your brain's interpretation of the sensory information it is receiving from your nose, your organs, and your digestive tract.

What if you picked up a carton of eggs, looked at the expiration date and realized that they had expired, but cracked an egg open and examined it carefully, trying to discern whether it looked "bad" just in case? Your ability to discern its current state is based on past experience with eggs and your cognitive interpretation of what eggs look like in various states. This is an example of top-down processing.

Imagine that you are working with a man named Alan and you ask him to pick up a 20-pound medicine ball that is sitting on the floor.

Alan has a history of low back pain and is worried about performing movements that will be injurious for his back. Alan looks at you and asks, "How do you want me to pick it up? Should I contract my abdominals? Do you want me to use my legs? Should I have my feet even?" How is Alan thinking about the movement?

His questions show that he is mostly thinking from a top-down perspective. He is trying to intellectualize the proper or best way to pick up the medicine ball so that he doesn't cause damage to his back (because somewhere along the line he was taught that picking things up might be harmful to the structures in his back). The thing is, when he performs the movement, the top-down processing might interfere with the bottom-up processing that occurs to coordinate joints and perform a specific action or movement based on a goal.

What if Alan drops the medicine ball accidentally and quickly bends down to pick it up without thinking about it? This would use more bottom-up processing because he is performing the movement in a habitual, more reflexive way. While managing movement using (mostly) top-down processing can interfere with natural coordination, when a person is sensitized or lacks movement options, top-down processing can be a useful way to bring awareness to unconscious habits and learn different movement strategies.

In an ideal world, movement would be taught using both top-down and bottom-up processing. For instance, I could ask Alan to pause, feel his feet against the ground, feel his hands against the weight, and focus on feeling the sensation of his feet as they press into the ground to stand up with the ball. Or I could ask Alan to initiate the movement by moving his pelvis towards the floor to get his torso closer to the ball, and then actively push his feet into the ground and move the pelvis away from the floor as he stands up. This is an example of using top-down processing to help organize the structure. I could give Alan key points that are (hopefully) slightly different than the ways he generally thinks about picking up the ball.

When you are learning a new skill, the first phase of learning is cognitive. This means you have to think about how to coordinate the joints to make the action happen. But at some point, as your neurons become more communicative and the pathways become more clear, the movement requires less conscious thought. This allows you to shift from thinking and more to feeling, focusing on the essence on the movement and what you feel as you perform it. In fact, when you try to interrupt this phase of learning by overthinking how you are performing the action, the skill will often get temporarily worse because you are disturbing the rapid communication of the neurons and asking them to communicate differently (Sternad, 2018).

Once Alan becomes comfortable with the act of picking up the ball, I could set three yoga blocks at different heights and ask Alan to pick up each of the blocks and set them back down. I could even make this more interesting by placing the blocks in varied relationships to Alan's body, so one block might be directly to his right, one might be to his left and back a little bit, and one might be in front of him and to his right. This particular action requires mostly bottom-up processing—too much conscious thought about how the movement should be performed will make the movement look less fluid and feel less coordinated.

The Physiology of the Fear Response

Fear prepares you for an immediate threat (real or imagined) through a brain/body process that causes you to respond in an innate or learned way. Fear learning happens when you are repeatedly exposed to a specific stimulus that you associate with danger. This leads to a conditioned behavior, like freezing (Keifer *et al.*, 2015).

If you heard a loud, rumbling sound at random intervals throughout the week, and the sound was accompanied by a stranger coming to your door, you might learn that each time you hear the noise, you should tense or jump, in preparation for the stranger's arrival. This is an example of fear learning and describes my nine-year-old dog Bob's relationship with the UPS truck—as soon as he hears it, he freezes, listening alertly, and then begins barking loudly.

If I exposed Bob to the sound of the UPS truck without the stranger coming to the door in a systematic way, and I used treats and threw his special red ball, eventually he would no longer associate the sound with the stranger. When the truck came back, he wouldn't freeze in anticipation, because the stimulus (truck sound) would be uncoupled from the thing he finds frightening. This is called fear extinction.

There are three well-established responses to fear: fight, flight, or freeze. Fight and flight are considered active coping strategies associated with an increase in SNS activation. Blood pressure, heart rate, respiration rate, and arousal increase as you prepare to expend energy to support your survival.

Immobilization or freezing are considered passive coping strategies, and occur when the threat can't be escaped. Much like "playing dead," the freeze response is associated with a decrease in blood pressure and a slowing of the heart rate. There is an increase in the neuroendocrine response as glucocorticoids flood the system and the hypothalamic pituitary adrenal axis (HPA axis) is activated. Freezing leads to conservation of energy and, like the fight or flight response, is situationally dependent. Which response is activated depends on the environment, probability of success, context, and individual.

The fear response originates in the amygdala, a small, almond-shaped set of neurons located in the brain's temporal lobe, and is part of the limbic system. The limbic system is composed of five sections: limbic cortex, hippocampal formation, amygdala, septal area, and hypothalamus.

The oldest part of the human brain is made up of the brainstem and the cerebellum. These structures allow us to live and breathe: the brainstem is responsible for managing automatic functions, including breathing, sleeping, and digestion, while the cerebellum is one of the brain areas responsible for motor output. The cerebellum is critical for limb movement and muscular contraction (Mottolese et al., 2013).

The limbic cortex, hypothalamus, and specific brainstem circuitry are the areas that control sympathetic and parasympathetic aspects of the ANS. The ANS controls a variety of functions, including heart rate, respiration rate, pupil constriction/dilation, and vasoconstriction/dilation (Tal & Devor, 2008). The different areas of the brain work together to maintain physiology and behavior.

In addition to heart rate and blood pressure regulation, the limbic system has a number of functions. It's involved with thought, experience, and senses. It helps you process things you are experiencing externally, such as paying attention to and experiencing emotions. It's involved with spatial memory, long-term memory, anxiety, fear conditioning, emotional memory, social cognition, and regulation of the ANS through hormone production and release. It may also be involved in your unconscious sense of safety—when the fear response is inhibited, opportunities open up for things like positive social experiences and engagement (Porges, 2007).

The neocortex is the most recently evolved portion of the brain and is sometimes referred to as the mammalian brain. In humans, it makes up about 80 percent of the brain size, has approximately 80 billion neurons, and is critical for allowing us to think and be consciously aware. It enables us to recognize faces, use tools, understand language, and understand social cues and interactions. It's what allows for cognition and what's enabling me to find the appropriate words to explain the concept to you. When we think of what makes us us, our thoughts and cognition from the neocortex are usually what we consider (Kaas, 2011).

Not only do all of these areas of the brain work together, allowing you to save energy through unconscious actions and enabling you to use conscious thought to converse, learn new things, and write books, but they are all also involved in the experience of movement. Movement is an expression of the input you receive from the world around you. You are constantly receiving and filtering all kinds of information—both internal information and external information (Dijkstra & Post, 2015). The movement that arises from that output represents your perception of that moment in time. Perception is influenced by many factors, as you will see in the upcoming sections.

The Physiology of Anxiety

I mentioned earlier that anxiety is rooted in uncertainty, while fear is a response to a perceived threat, either real or imagined. To experience anxiety is to feel a lack of control, a sense that the future holds potentially detrimental experiences that can't be altered (Steimer, 2002).

Remember my sister and client from the beginning of the chapter? Both were afraid of serious illnesses. Their fear wasn't rooted in a perceived threat, like a potentially dangerous situation, or actually feeling unwell: they were both afraid of what could happen *if*, not what could happen *because*.

The development of anxiety is dependent on at least two sets of factors: the influence of the environment and genetics. How we cope and experience the world is a complicated interplay between what we are exposed to (people, experiences, living quarters, having basic needs met) and our biology. Both fear-related active coping and anxiety cause activation of the ANS; however, researchers have proposed that feelings of anxiety are organized in the locus coeruleus (LC), a tiny cell structure referred to as a nucleus that is located in the brainstem and innervates the cerebral cortex (Samuels & Szabadi, 2008). It's the largest group of neurons that releases the neurotransmitter norepinephrine in the CNS and correlates closely with arousal levels, which keep you awake and alert. The hormone and neurotransmitter that makes you feel awake and alert, norepinephrine, is produced by the noradrenergic neurons (Plummer *et al.*, 2017).

Neurotransmitters: An Overview

Hormones are made in specific areas. They are then transmitted to nerve cells via neurotransmitters. If the cell membrane is able to receive the hormone, the hormone will penetrate the cell, causing specific genes to activate. This response results in a behavior of some sort, whether it's an increase in heart rate, the inability to fall asleep, or the movement of a leg. We are essentially one large chemistry experiment, with inputs coming from both inside and outside of us that influence which genes are expressed and which aren't.

Because the LC plays such a pivotal (and far-reaching) role in the activation of the SNS, LC activation leads to a decrease in PSNS activity. Basically, long-term LC activation throws the nervous system off balance, tipping activity in favor of more alert, wakeful behavior (if you've ever wondered why the experience of anxiety makes it difficult to sleep, you can blame LC activation).

Another physiological factor that occurs during the presence of anxiety is altered activity of the HPA axis. When something stressful happens, whether it's physical or psychological, it activates the HPA axis. The result? The hypothalamus releases corticotropin-releasing factor (CRF), which causes the pituitary gland to release adrenocorticotropic hormone (ACTH). ACTH travels to the adrenal gland, where it binds to receptors, and boom...cortisol is released! Cortisol is commonly thought of as the stress hormone, and influences mood and behavior in a number of ways (Faravelli *et al.*, 2012).

Cortisol isn't bad; in fact, its release follows our circadian rhythms. When you wake up, cortisol levels are low, which is why you feel groggy and content to stay in bed a little longer. Cortisol levels peak about 30 minutes after waking up. You are energetic, are able to focus, and don't feel sleepy at all. As the day wears on, cortisol levels slowly decline (which is perhaps why you feel sleepy around 3:00 p.m.—your cortisol levels have waned and with them, your arousal levels). This, of course, isn't set in stone—there are individual differences, and this arc can vary, but it does tend to be the general trend.

Glucocorticoid receptors, the receptors for cortisol, are found in almost every cell of the human body. This means cortisol affects muscles, heart rate, breathing, hormones, and the nervous system (Thau & Sharma, 2019). It controls the stress response (the presence of cortisol actually inhibits the hormones that trigger production of cortisol in healthy individuals), and when it is released because of a threatening situation, it keeps you alert and awake. Cortisol increases the availability of blood glucose to the brain, promoting a variety of metabolic shifts, such as increasing gluconeogenesis and decreasing glycogen synthesis. Gluconeogenesis is the generation of glucose (a simple sugar used in metabolism) from non-carbohydrate substrates. Glycogen synthesis is the conversion of glucose to glycogen in the liver, which is needed for glycogen storage.

This all means that cortisol plays a role in metabolism. It is also critical for the maintenance of daily arousal and function.

As we move forward and you learn about different exercise and movement interventions for mental health, you may begin to realize that different times of day work best for different movement interventions. For instance, if the anxious person, who already has high levels of cortisol in their body, wants to begin a restorative practice, should the person do that in the morning or the evening? Probably later in the day when their cortisol levels are lower. This will make it easier for them to feel a sense of relaxation.

What if you are working with someone who describes themselves as low energy, has trouble staying motivated, and finds exercise difficult? What would be the best movement intervention and time of day for that individual? Probably something that will stimulate cortisol production, like cardiovascular exercise or an exercise program that increases heart rate periodically throughout the session. And maybe if this were done in the morning, one to two hours after the person got up, it would keep that individual's cortisol levels slightly higher for longer throughout the day and make them feel better.

One of the markers of a healthy stress response is resilience; part of resilience is adaptability. We will discuss this further in Chapter 3.

Early childhood stress can also cause an alteration in the stress response that lasts throughout adulthood. Being separated from one's mother during infancy or childhood abuse and neglect are associated with long-term changes in brain circuity and the regulation of stress reactivity, mood, and behavior (Faravelli *et al.*, 2012). It is worth noting that a history of anxiety and depression may be indicative of long-term trauma. You may find that the most effective movement interventions for long-term trauma aren't always the same as the ones that work best for people with just anxiety or just depression.

In people struggling with major depressive disorder, a mental health disorder that will affect 20 percent of people at some point in their lives and is difficult to treat pharmaceutically, the cells that inhibit production of glucocorticoids are less sensitive. This results in the production of more cortisol, leading to the impairment of working memory and a heart that is more reactive to stress (Menke, 2019). Fortunately, exercise interventions can help regulate and restore the HPA axis. You will learn more about how this works in Chapter 2 when we explore the effects of aerobic exercise on mental health.

The Physiology of Stress

Stress is defined physiologically as a series of events consisting of a stimulus (stressor) that causes a reaction in the brain (stress perception), activating a physiological stress response. Put more simply: stressor → stress perception → stress response (Dhabhar, 2018).

Hans Selye, an endocrinologist who is often considered the "father of stress research," was the first to identify the effects of chronic stress as a contributing factor to unspecified symptoms and illness. He proposed that the chronic stress response occurs in three phases: the alarm phase, the resistance stage, and the exhaustion stage. He linked this to hyperactivity of the adrenal system, lymphatic atrophy, and peptic ulcers (Tan & Yip, 2018).

The lymphatic system is a vascular system that transports immune cells and antigens and prevents swelling in the tissues (Moore & Bertram, 2018). Peptic ulcers are believed to be an acid-driven disease occurring in both the gastric and duodenal areas of the intestinal system. They are difficult to treat and are believed to be caused by a variety of factors, including chronic stress.

Selye is also credited with coining the term "eustress," which means the stressor is perceived as something pleasant as opposed to harmful. It has been proposed that short-term stress enhances immune function and can have beneficial effects on the brain, body, and health (Dhabhar, 2018). This differs from Selye's belief that eustress, though perceived as pleasant, behaves from a physiological standpoint like distress and can cause damage. Curiously, though Selye viewed his work as leisure, he was, by all accounts, a workaholic—he authored more than 40 books and 1600 scientific articles. It could be argued that someone who transforms his home into the International Institute of Stress is an example of using eustress to energize and maintain a high level of productivity (Tan & Yip, 2018). Did he experience damaging effects to his immune system because of his devotion to his work? It's impossible to know, but I suspect there is little he would change about his professional life if he were still alive today.

All of this is to say that stress is an inevitable aspect of life. I was at a lecture on stress recently where the speaker, a Stanford professor and author, asked the audience to reflect on what gave us meaning and purpose. After giving us time to share our responses with each other, she asked, "Does the thing that gives you meaning and purpose ever cause you stress?"

Almost every hand in the room went up as we laughed, recognizing that things we care deeply about aren't free from stress. The goal isn't to have a stress-free life. Rather, it's to view stress as a worthwhile challenge and a way to harness energy, and to use that energy to support our situation and to rely on the support of, and connect with, others through our experience.

As you will see in subsequent chapters, exercise is a form of stress—one that requires energy, is temporarily challenging, and results in more strength. The realizations that discomfort is temporary, that the body is strong, adaptable, and capable of learning, and that the proper social support can alter our experience affect more than just our physical well-being. These lessons translate into our emotional processing and how we experience the world.

Depression

Depression disorders are not the antithesis of anxiety disorders. In fact, they often co-exist, wreaking havoc on a person's emotional well-being.

Depression is characterized by a low, sad, or depressed mood and a loss of interest in activities that were previously pleasurable. Characters such as Eeyore from *Winnie the Pooh* regularly have a more depressed outlook on life. Even Calvin from the comic strip *Calvin and Hobbes* has days where his most favorite rocket ship underpants don't work to make him feel better.

It's okay to have an off day once in a while. But when the off days happen more often than not, or when weeks go by and you haven't once smiled, it's no longer a case of rocket underpants not helping. Physical symptoms of depression include changes in appetite and weight, sleep trouble (sleeping more or less than normal), issues with motor control and coordination, and fatigue (*Primary Care Companion to the Journal of Clinical Psychiatry*, 2008). The development of major depressive disorder is attributed partially to genetic factors (experts think 30–40 percent), leaving 60–70 percent of the variance being due to individualized environmental effects (Hasler, 2010). Examples include adverse events in childhood and recent stress due to low social support, marital problems, and lifetime trauma (*ibid.*). Women generally show greater stress responsiveness to the physiological release of stress hormones than men, consistent with the larger incidences of depression in women.

When the HPA axis is affected during childhood trauma, the secretion of the stress hormones is altered. Interestingly, most individuals struggling with major depressive disorder don't appear to have HPA-axis dysfunction. What does appear to be altered is serotonin, also known as the happiness hormone, which is responsible for a number of behaviors, like eating, sleep, mood, perception, and reward (Frazer & Hensler, 1999; Berger *et al.*, 2018). The release of serotonin is controlled by the hypothalamus. Fortunately, one of the ways to increase serotonin also happens to be the topic of this book: exercise (Kang & So, 2018).

Unfortunately, depression and anxiety are often under-diagnosed. It's common for primary care physicians to see patients with somatic complaints who also display symptoms related to anxiety or depression (Haftgoli *et al.*, 2010). Only if a medical provider probes deeper, asking questions about psychological well-being, is mental health assessed. This, of course, requires treatment of the person, not the symptoms. *Of course, as movement professionals, we aren't in a position to diagnose or assert opinions regarding a client's mental health; however, understanding the symptoms makes it easier for you to know when you should suggest that clients talk to their doctors or healthcare providers.*

Often when people think of depression, they think of major depressive disorder, which is severe and potentially life threatening. According to the DSM-5 (American Psychiatric Association, 2013), if you have five or more of the following symptoms, you may have major depressive disorder:

- You are depressed most of the day, most days of the week.
- You aren't interested in/don't get pleasure from activities during the day.
- You gain or lose a lot of weight or you have a significant increase or decrease in your appetite.
- Your thoughts are slow and you are moving less.
- You are extremely tired or don't have energy during the day.
- You feel guilty or worthless on a daily basis.
- You struggle to think, concentrate, or make decisions.
- You have regular thoughts of death or suicide.

Another form of depression, persistent depressive disorder, is milder and chronic in nature. One of the criteria for diagnosis is a depressed mood for at least two years. Risk factors for persistent depressive disorder include genetics, trauma, low sense of self-worth, and high-anxiety states (Patel & Rose, 2019). Persistent depressive disorder is associated with greater severity of anxiety and somatic symptoms than major depressive disorder and used to be called "dysthymia" (the term was first used in relation to psychiatry by C. F. Fleming in 1844 and comes from the Greek word *dusthumia*, which means despondency or despair).

Trauma

Me: "What was the birth of your son like?"
Client: "I almost bled to death. I don't remember much, really, it all happened so fast."

Trauma is defined as "actual or threatened death, serious injury, or sexual violence" (Center for Substance Abuse Treatment (US), 2014a). Psychosocial stressors, like divorce or job loss, are not considered to be trauma in this definition. Post-traumatic stress disorder (PTSD) is a clinical diagnosis that includes experiencing trauma directly, witnessing others experience trauma, indirect exposure to trauma through a family member's experience, or repeated or extreme exposure to the details of traumatic events. The latter includes professions like forensic child abuse investigators or military mortuary workers.

Not everyone who experiences trauma will display criteria associated with PTSD. In fact, many people exhibit responses consistent with resiliency or that are brief and in line with individual coping skills (Center for Substance Abuse Treatment (US), 2014b). How trauma is processed is based on a number of factors, including past experience, support systems, and life skills. Recent research suggests that talking about the traumatic event and the emotions surrounding it isn't necessarily required for a healthy psychological response. Healthy coping is demonstrated by the ability to continue daily activities, regulate emotions, maintain self-esteem, and maintain social connection. Coping strategies are specific to the individual, with many different styles of coping leading to healthy outcomes.

When someone is unable to cope with trauma in a psychologically healthy way and their symptoms are consistent with PTSD, a number of neuroreceptors are affected, including adrenoreceptors and serotonergic receptors, both of which are regulated by aspects of the limbic system. Dysregulation of these receptors leads to unhealthy stress and fear-related responses, including difficulties with emotional process and behavioral regulation (Bailey *et al.*, 2013). Research also suggests that PTSD is linked to dysregulation of the HPA axis, leading to an increase in corticotropin-releasing factor (CRF), which is linked to higher levels of cortisol.

At this point, the mechanisms behind the physiology should be feeling slightly more familiar even if you are getting bogged down by the neuroscience. Stressful event happens. Hormones are released in an effort to mitigate the stressor. In most situations, the individual returns to baseline. In some situations, baseline is disrupted, and things become dysregulated.

It should come as no surprise, then, that PTSD is often comorbid with anxiety and depression; in fact, PTSD is considered by some researchers to be predictive of other mental health disorders. Conversely, anxiety and depression are not necessarily predictive of PTSD

(Ginzburg *et al.*, 2010). The increase in SNS activity that occurs with PTSD throws off ANS balance, resulting in a higher risk of hypertension and cardiovascular disease.

A recent study (Fonkoue *et al.*, 2020) compared inflammatory and cardiovascular markers between three groups of military veterans: 28 with severe PTSD, 16 with moderate PTSD, and 26 controls. Subjects were asked to perform mental math problems for three minutes while being urged to answer accurately and faster. This is a test that is often used in clinical settings because it is considered mentally stressful (imagine someone yelling out math problems for you to do in your head and then shouting, "You need to answer faster! Look at the clock," for three minutes—it makes me feel slightly anxious just thinking about it).

A number of measurements were performed while subjects were working through this equivalent of a mental gymnastics performance. Though the mental math led to similar increases in SNS activity between the groups, individuals with severe PTSD exhibited higher inflammation, impaired baroreflex[1] sensitivity, a higher likelihood of high resting heart rate, and higher withdrawal of the PSNS at the onset of the mentally stressful situation than the controls. This shows that emotional health directly affects physiological health.

"Homeostasis," a term that describes how physiological and behavioral responses occur in a coordinated way to stabilize or maintain specific physiological parameters like blood pressure and blood sugar, can be thought of as our physiological balance. Just like physical stability can be thought of as the ability to recover from an outside perturbation and can be achieved in many ways, eliminating the idea that any one posture is perfect, a perfect physiological balance point is elusive—an impossibility because there are always perturbations acting upon us and we are in a perpetual state of change, even if it's seemingly imperceptible.

Allostasis, a model first coined by Peter Sterling and Joseph Ayer in 1988 (Ramsay & Woods, 2014), is defined as achieving stability through change. Allostasis is based on three main principles (*ibid.*):

- If we want to regulate our internal state efficiently, the regulation is anticipatory. We learn from past events and anticipate the

---

1 Baroreflex controls heart rate and resistance of the peripheral arteries. It is the fastest way to regulate acute blood pressure. Baroreflex sensitivity refers to how much control the baroreflex has on heart rate.

appropriate neurological response before the event happens. If you eat lunch at noon every day, you will be ready, both physiologically and emotionally, for food at noon regardless of the situation.

- The body doesn't have strict, unchanging set points; regulated values can and should change to cope with the demands presented by the environment. If you move to a place that is hot and humid, you will sweat sooner when running than in a place that is cool and dry (Romanovsky, 2018). If you move to a place that is cool and dry, once you've acclimated you will no longer sweat.
- A central command center in the brain activates and deactivates multiple responses, influencing regulated variables in order to reach the most energy-efficient compromises to maintain optimal regulation.

When there is an underlying sense of constant fear, when we feel depressed, or when a traumatic event occurs, our system works hard to maintain optimal functioning by activating responses that alter physiology and affect behavior. This shift can cause a cascade of events and impact several areas of physical health and well-being. However, because we are an organism that is capable of learning, we have the power to shift things in a different direction. Exercise and movement can alter one aspect of our physiology that in turn affects another. If you view the entire self as capable of learning and, therefore, capable of change, this mindset will affect not only how you teach, but also how your clients receive your words and experience your work. The more you believe people can change, the more likely the person in front of you will believe it, too.

Understanding how mental health disorders, specifically anxiety, depression, and PTSD, can impact biology and physiology makes it more clear how a person's mental health affects the entire person. The parallels between mental well-being and physical well-being are palpable, and they are intertwined in such a way that when you work with people in a movement setting, you are creating opportunities to influence the whole person. As you will see throughout the book, how you show up and are present is an important aspect to enabling clients to find an access point for movement to transcend the physical benefits. We are a species whose well-being is multi-faceted and is determined by the physical body, mental health, and our interactions with others.

It's important to remember that beginning anything new is both scary and exciting. Your new clients don't know what to expect from their first meeting. The type of environment you create can put people at ease, allowing them to feel safe and engage with you, ultimately facilitating their ability to try new movements and skills so they can build strength and confidence.

References

American Psychiatric Association (2013). Diagnostic and Statistical Manual of Mental Disorders. 5th edition. https://doi.org/10.1176/appi.books.9780890425596.

Bailey C.R., Cordell E., Sobin S.M., & Neumeister A. (2013). Recent progress in understanding the pathophysiology of post-traumatic stress disorder: Implications for targeted pharmacological treatment. CNS Drugs, 27(3), 221-232.

Barral J.-P., & Croibier A. (2009). Chapter 11: Optic Nerve, 73-89. In: Manual Therapy for the Cranial Nerves. Cambridge, MA: Elsevier.

Berger M., Gray J.A., & Roth B.L. (2018). The expanded biology of serotonin. Annual Review of Medicine, 60, 355-366.

Bordoni B., Reed R.R., Taci P., & Varacallo M. (2020). Neuroanatomy, cranial nerve 11 (accessory). In: Statpearls [Internet]. Treasure Island, FL: Statpearls Publishing.

Center for Substance Abuse Treatment (US) (2014a). Exhibit 1.3-4, DSM-5 Diagnostic Criterial for PTSD. In: Trauma-Informed Care in Behavioral Health Services. Rockville, MD: Substance Abuse and Mental Health Services Administration (US). Treatment Improvement Protocol (TIP) Series, No. 57.

Center for Substance Abuse Treatment (US) (2014b). Chapter 3: Understanding the Impact of Trauma. In: Trauma-Informed Care in Behavioral Health Services. Rockville, MD: Substance Abuse and Mental Health Services Administration (US). Treatment Improvement Protocol (TIP) Series, No. 57.

Cohodes E.M., & Gee D.G. (2017). Developmental neurobiology of anxiety and related disorders. Oxford Research Encyclopedia, Neuroscience, 1-28.

Cuevas J. (2007). The somatic nervous system. XPharm: The Comprehensive Pharmacology Reference, 1-13.

Cuevas J. (2011). The peripheral nervous system. Xpharm: The Comprehensive Pharmacological Reference, 1-2.

Dhabhar F.S. (2018). The short-term stress response: Mother nature's mechanism for enhancing protection and performance under conditions of threat, challenge, and opportunity. Frontiers in Neuroendocrinology, 49, 175-192.

Dijkstra K., & Post L. (2015). Mechanisms of embodiments. Frontiers in Psychology, 6, 1525.

Faravelli C., Sauro C.L., Godini L., Lelli L., Benni L., et al. (2012). Childhood stressful events, HPA axis and anxiety disorders. World Journal of Psychiatry, 2(1), 13-25.

Felton D., O'Banion M., & Maida M. (2016). Brain Stem and Cerebellum. In: Netter's Atlas of Neuroscience. 3rd edition. Philadelphia, PA: Elsevier.

Fischer D.B., & Truog R.D. (2015). What is a reflex? A guide for understanding disorders of consciousness. Neurology, 85(6), 543-548.

Fonkoue I.T., Marvar P.J., Nordholm S., Li Y., Kankam M.L., *et al.* (2020). Symptom severity impacts sympathetic dysregulation and inflammation in post traumatic stress disorder. Brain Behavior and Immunology, 83, 260-269.

Frazer A., & Hensler J.G. (1999). Serotonin Involvement in Physiological Function and Behavior. In: Siegel G.J., Agranoff B.W., Albers R.W., Fisher S.K., & Uhler M.D. (eds) Basic Neurochemistry: Molecular, Cellular and Medical Aspects. 6th edition. Philadelphia, PA: Lippincott-Raven.

Ginzburg K., Ein-Dor T., & Solomon Z. (2010). Comorbidity of post traumatic stress disorder, anxiety and depression: A 20 year longitudinal study of war veterans. Journal of Affective Disorder, 123(1-3), 249-257.

Haftgoli N., Favrat B., Verdon F., Vaucher P., *et al.* (2010). Patients presenting with somatic complaints in general practice: Depression, anxiety and somatic disorders are frequent and associated with psychosocial stressors. BMC Family Practice, 11(67).

Hasler G. (2010). Pathophysiology of depression: Do we have solid evidence of interest to clinicians? World Psychiatry, 9(3), 155-161.

Kaas J.H. (2011). Neocortex in early mammals and its subsequent variations. New Perspectives on Neurobehavioral Evolution, 1225(1), 28-36.

Kang S.H., & So W.Y. (2018). Effect of competitive and non-competitive exercise on serotonin levels in adolescents with various levels of internet gaming addiction. Iranian Journal of Public Health, 47(7), 1047-1049.

Keifer O.P., Hurt R.C., Ressler K.J., & Marvar P.J. (2015). The physiology of fear: Reconceptualizing the role of the central amygdala in fear learning. Physiology (Bethesda), 30(5), 898-401.

Kenny B.J., & Bordoni B. (2019). Neuroanatomy, cranial nerve 10 (vagus nerve). In: Statpearls [Internet]. Treasure Island, FL: Statpearls Publishing.

Knight L.K., & Depue B.E. (2019). New frontiers in anxiety research: The translational potential of the bed nucleus of the stria terminals. Frontiers in Psychiatry, 10, 510.

Menke A. (2019). Is the HPA axis as target for depression outdated, or is there new hope? Frontiers in Psychiatry, 10, 101.

Moore Jr. J.E., & Bertram C.D. (2018). Lymphatic system flows. Annual Review of Fluid Mechanics, 50, 459-482.

Morell P., & Quarles R.H. (1999). The Myelin Sheath. In: Siegel G.J., Agranoff B.W., Albers R.W., Fisher S.K., & Uhler M.D (eds) Basic Neurochemistry: Molecular, Cellular and Medical Aspects. 6th edition. Philadelphia, PA: Lippincott-Raven.

Mottolese C., Richard N., Harquel S., Szathmari A., Sirigu A., & Desmurget M. (2013). Mapping motor representation in the human cerebellum. Brain: A Journal of Neurology, 136(1), 330-342.

Nogradi A., & Vrbova G. (2000–2013). Anatomy and Physiology of the Spinal Cord. In: Madame Curie Bioscience Database [Internet]. Austin, TX: Landes Bioscience.

Patel R.K., & Rose G.M. (2019). Persistent depressive disorder (dysthymia). In: StatPearls [Internet]. Treasure Island, FL: StatPearls Publishing.

Plummer N.W., Scappini E.L., Smith K.G., Tucker C.J., & Jensen P. (2017). Two subpopulations of noradrenergic neurons in the locus coeruleus complex distinguished by the expression of the dorsal neural tube marker Pax7. Frontiers in Neuroanatomy, 60, 11.

Porges S. (2007). The polyvagal perspective. Biological Psychology, 74(2), 116-143.

Primary Care Companion to the Journal of Clinical Psychiatry (2008). Treating depression and anxiety in primary care. Primary Care Companion to the Journal of Clinical Psychiatry, 10(2), 145-152.

Ramsay D.S., & Woods S.C. (2014). Clarifying the roles of homeostasis and allostasis in physiological regulation. Psychology Review, 121(2), 225-247.

Rauss K., & Pourtois G. (2013). What is bottom-up and what is top-down predictive coding? Frontiers in Psychology, 276.

Rea P. (2014). Clinical Anatomy of the Cranial Nerves. Cambridge, MA: Elsevier.

Romano N., Federici M., & Castaldi A. (2019). Imaging of cranial nerves: A pictorial overview. Insights Imaging, 10, 33

Romanovsky A.A. (2018). Thermoregulation: From Basic Neuroscience to Clinical Neurology, Part II. Boston, MA: Elsevier.

Samuels E.R., & Szabadi E. (2008). Functional neuroanatomy of the noradrenergic locus coeruleus: Its roles in the regulation of arousal and autonomic function part I: principles of functional organisation. Current Neuropharmacology, 6(3), 235-253.

Snyder J.M., Hagan C.E., Bolon B., & Keene C.D. (2018). Chapter 20: Nervous System. In: Treating P.M., Dintzis S.M., & Montine K.S. (eds) Comparative Anatomy and Histology: A Mouse, Rat, and Human Atlas. 2nd edition. Cambridge, MA: Elsevier.

Sonne J., & Lopez-Ojeda W. (2019). Neuroanatomy, cranial nerve. In: Statpearls [Internet]. Treasure Island, FL: Statpearls Publishing.

Steimer T. (2002). The biology of fear- and anxiety-related behaviors. Dialogues in Clinical Neuroscience, 4(3), 231-249.

Sternad D. (2018). It's not (only) the mean that matters: Variability, noise and exploration in motor learning. Current Opinions in Behavioral Science, 20, 183-195.

Susuki K. (2010). Myelin: A specialized membrane for cell communication. Nature Education, 3(9), 59.

Tal M. & Devor M. (2008). Chapter 2: Anatomy and Neurophysiology of Orofacial Pain. In: Share Y., & Benoliel R. (eds) Orofacial Pain and Headache. Boston, MA: Elsevier Health Sciences.

Tan S.Y., & Yip A. (2018). Hans Selye (1907-1982): Founder of the stress theory. Singapore Medical Journal, 59(4), 170-171.

Thau L., & Sharma S. (2019). Physiology, cortisol. In: Statpearls [Internet]. Treasure Island, FL: Statpearls Publishing.

CHAPTER 2

Why Cardiovascular Activity?

My sister called me recently to let me know she was planning on using the Peloton bike she purchased a year ago on a regular basis. "The kids are finally sleeping in the early mornings and I feel so much less anxious after I exercise."

Cardiovascular, or aerobic, activity isn't only good for anxiety, it can also improve symptoms of depression and PTSD. There is something about rhythmic, sustained movement that improves the health of the entire system, from the heart and lungs to the brain.

The word "endurance" comes from the French word *endurer*, which means to make hard. Endurance is the ability to withstand difficult situations. When we endure, we survive. We overcome the difficulties presented to us and persevere.

People begin an exercise program for many reasons and are generally motivated by either extrinsic or intrinsic factors. You know when someone comes to you and says they want to lose weight? That's an extrinsic factor. What about the person who simply wants to feel better, who wants a sense of control over their emotions? That person is motivated by an intrinsic factor.

Extrinsic factors include the desire to change how others perceive you, to change a physiological measurement (like weight, inches, or blood pressure), or to look a certain way. Intrinsic factors often include the desire to feel different, to improve confidence, and/or to feel calmer.

When someone is motivated to begin an exercise program by extrinsic factors, it's more difficult to maintain momentum when things get tedious or hard. It may also make it difficult to find the appropriate starting place. One of the biggest barriers to sustaining an exercise program is doing too much too soon. This leads to excessive soreness or, worse, injury.

You can help someone identify the appropriate starting point for exercise by figuring out what they want to accomplish. What the individual is motivated by will directly influence how you suggest that they approach beginning an exercise program. If someone wants to lose ten pounds in five weeks, the exercise intervention used may feel doable for the five weeks, allowing the individual to push through discomfort and soreness, but it's not likely to be sustainable for the duration of their life. Helping the client or patient understand that they are more than likely not going to be creating a lifelong habit because they are looking at exercise as a short-term fix can help manage the their expectations about what will happen after the goal is accomplished.

If goals are fueled by a desire to reduce anxiety symptoms and feel calmer, more stable, and stronger, exercise becomes a long-term intervention instead of a short-term fix. This mindset makes it easier to view exercise as a lifestyle choice, an aspect of the day that is important not only because of an arbitrary number, but also because of its impact on emotional and physical well-being.

The downfall of intrinsic goals is that it can take longer for the benefits to become obvious. They happen slowly, gradually seeping into a person's life until the individual realizes that they have changed on some fundamental level. They are reacting to things differently, they feel more balanced, and they have more control and a greater sense of their body.

My sister has exercised enough throughout her life to know that when she does regular cardiovascular activity, she sleeps better, is less reactive, and doesn't fall into specific thought patterns. She prefers not feeling anxious to feeling anxious, so prioritizing exercise is important to her. Asking people about their long-term goals for beginning a walking or running program, riding the Peloton regularly, or buying the latest rowing machine can help them clarify their why. Asking them to reflect on how they feel once they begin a regular aerobic exercise program can provide perspective about changes that go beyond extrinsic factors.

The Role of Breath

When someone experiences feelings of worry or anxiousness, breathing strategies change. During relaxed breathing, the breath is slower and fuller. The inhale expands the lungs and causes the diaphragm, which looks like an upside-down parachute, to contract. When the diaphragm contracts, the parachute fills, moves down, and causes the viscera (organs) to descend. This is why the stomach expands on the inhale—the diaphragm causes a shift in the placement of the organs. (The lungs cause the ribs to expand as well, so breathing is actually a subtle, total-body movement.) The pelvic floor (a common name for the muscles that make up the inside base of the pelvis) moves down as well, causing the muscles of the pelvic floor to relax.

During the exhale, everything reverses. The pelvic floor contracts and moves up, the organs shift as the stomach softens, and the diaphragm passively relaxes and moves up as carbon dioxide leaves the lungs and is expelled in the air. The inhale and exhale are soft, requiring no obvious muscular contraction, and the exhale is longer than the inhale.

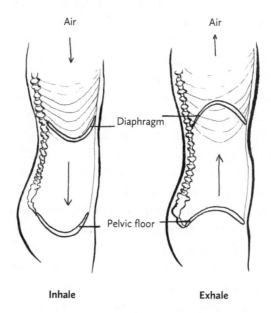

RESPIRATION AND PELVIC FLOOR

When a person feels anxious, instead of the inhale traveling down, the breath stays up in the chest. When the breath stays up, the chest and neck muscles contract and relax with each inhale and exhale. This makes the breath more shallow and can result in feeling like you aren't quite getting enough air. Since air is an important part of life, this causes the respiration rate to increase. The inhales and exhales might become even, affecting heart rate variability (which we will discuss in a moment), or the individual may adopt a strategy of breath holding, as though they were saving the inhale, protecting the air that enters the lungs, and using it to keep the torso upright and stable.

There are shifts in our day-to-day life that require the breathing rate to change subtly in order to match the amount of energy required to perform various tasks. While breathing can be controlled, for reasons we will discuss later, that isn't always the best initial choice for anxious individuals. Another way to regulate breath is through cardiovascular exercise (also called CV exercise).

During sustained aerobic activity, the breathing rate increases to accommodate the extra oxygen needed for the muscles to work and to clear the excess metabolic waste (also known as carbon dioxide) that is being produced by the muscles (Your Lungs and Exercise, 2016). Interesting fact: if you tried to exhale all of the air out of your lungs, assuming your lungs are healthy, there would still be air left over. This air is referred to as the residual volume, and it keeps the alveoli (tiny air sacs inside the lungs that enable gas to be exchanged rapidly) open (Lofrese & Lappin, 2019). This means even when someone feels out of breath, they still have air in the lungs that's keeping everything working.

When sustained aerobic exercise is performed at a high enough intensity, the respiration rate remains slightly elevated even after the bout of exercise has ended. This may be because the body continues working at a slightly more elevated rate after exercise is over, so muscles still need extra oxygen to deal with the amount of work. It's like if you set the oven to 350 degrees for 30 minutes; even after you've removed the cookies and turned the oven off, it will still give off heat for a while until it cools down. When exercise ends, it takes the body time to cool off, which requires energy. How much time it takes depends on how high you "turned the oven up" and for how long—it would take longer to return to your resting respiration rate if you were climbing steep stairs for two hours than if you went for a leisurely 20-minute walk on flat ground. Excess post-exercise oxygen consumption (EPOC) provides the necessary fuel; your breath provides the extra oxygen (Laforgia *et al.*, 2006).

Eventually, respiration returns to normal after the exercise bout. In fact, if you asked someone to gauge their respiration rate before exercising, during exercise, and an hour after exercise, their respiration rate an hour after exercise might feel slower than it did before exercise. Work makes the contrast to rest sharper, altering perception.

If someone hasn't done more than walk across the parking lot from the car to their office in years, then the increase in breathing rate and the burning sensation in their lungs they experience the first time they go for a fast walk up the hill near their house may make them think the walk is a bad idea.

The good news is the burning sensation in the lungs and the rapid breathing will improve with practice. That's because the lungs and heart, like any muscle in the body, become stronger and more efficient with use; this newfound strength and ease requires less oxygen, allowing the breath to slow and the cardiovascular system to work less hard.

Recently, I saw a client who has been working with me regularly for a while. She's strong, comfortable in a variety of positions, and doesn't have any pain or discomfort anywhere. She went hiking for the first time in a year: "My chest felt heavy, like it was burning."

"Have you been walking regularly?

"No. I haven't made the time for it."

I laughed and told her the only solution for strengthening the lungs was to use the lungs on a regular basis. "I don't do that part for you," I told her.

The Heart

If you were told that in ten minutes, you were going to stand up in front of 100 medical professionals and give a lecture on how aerobic exercise impacts mental health, how would you feel?

Unless this is your area of expertise, you would probably notice a few things happening. You may feel your jaw and neck clench. You might have difficulty swallowing. Your muscles may tense up, and you may suddenly feel your heart beating quickly, as if it were going to jump out of your chest.

These are normal sensations related to anxiety. They are also normal sensations related to any sort of stress, whether it's short term or long term. The heartbeat, which during rest isn't noticeable at all unless you think about it, can become remarkably loud when you feel emotionally amped up. The ability to observe physiological sensations, such as the heart rate and the breath, is called interoception.

Interoception can be defined as the perception of bodily sensations. Things like whether you are full or hungry, if you are experiencing discomfort in your abdomen, or how fast you are breathing are all sensations related to interoceptive awareness. Interoception is largely unconscious. When you are consciously aware of your interoceptive state, how you interpret those interoceptive signals can influence your emotional state (Price & Hooven, 2018).

Think about the last time you were really nervous about something, maybe a job interview or big social engagement. Did you find yourself uninterested in food in the hour leading up to the interview or party, even though it was time for a meal? Your lack of hunger might not be related to a physiological response; rather, your emotional state is likely contributing to the lack of physiological desire to eat. The emotions and body are interconnected, which means our internal signals are heavily influenced by both our physical and emotional states in the immediate moment. Understanding this interconnectedness makes it easier to observe physical responses in a less judgmental way.

How accurately you can discern your level of cardiovascular arousal may correlate with emotional regulation. For example, if your heart rate elevates slightly but your perception is that it has suddenly increased significantly, this mismatch between what is happening and what you perceive will change how you respond to it. Perceiving that your heart rate is significantly elevated when it isn't may cause shortness of breath and a sensation of panic, just like getting ready to walk into a room full of people you don't know may cause you to lose your appetite (Garfinkle et al., 2016). Your panicked response and emotional reaction will cause the heart rate to elevate more, creating a self-fulfilling prophecy of an inaccurate perception causing an overreaction throughout the SNS.

During the day, there are all kinds of fluctuations that occur in your physiological state. Those things that require more energy, and thus, more oxygen, cause you to breathe faster and the heart to beat faster, like when you are rushing out of the house in the morning to drop the kids off before the school bell so you can get to your 9:00 a.m. meeting without looking like you just rolled out of bed.

On the other hand, when you are staring at emails at 2:00 p.m. and you feel your eyes get heavy and are tempted to close the door, lie down, and take a nap, your breathing and heart rate are slower. These fluctuations are mostly unconscious, unless you consciously focus once in a while on what you are experiencing. In fact, heart rate variability, which refers to fluctuations in heart rate, is considered an indicator of cardiovascular health; it's also been linked to balance between the PSNS and SNS (West & Turalska, 2019, Cornelissen *et al.*, 2010).

Conveniently, the heart is an organ that is controlled by the ANS and is influenced by breath, which is also controlled (mostly) by the ANS (Sasaki & Maruyama, 2014). The inhale speeds the heart rate up; the exhale slows it down. The inhale correlates with SNS activity and the exhale correlates with PSNS activity. This means every time you breathe you are influencing your heart rate and your nervous system, which ultimately influences how you feel.

It's probably no surprise that a number of things influence arousal states and that brain arousal affects all aspects of human behavior (Huang *et al.*, 2018). Factors like your genetics, how safe you feel, your ability to self-regulate, and how much you slept last night all influence your baseline level of arousal. Learning to gauge accurately how you feel and notice what influences your baseline can impact other areas of your life in a profound way.

One of the goals of aerobic exercise is to elevate the heart rate for a sustained period of time. The elevated heart rate increases arousal, which means the behavior (the aerobic activity) creates the arousal state. SNS activity increases, heart rate increases, and respiration rate increases. You become more alert and focused. The amount of arousal corresponds to both the intensity of the exercise and how adapted you are to the stimulus. I run a relatively hilly four to seven miles, three days a week. I have been doing this for over two decades and, while my heart rate and breathing do elevate, I barely notice it. I am habituated to the speed and terrain over which I run.

If I were to go running with the local marathon runners, many of whom not only post times that qualify for the Boston Marathon but also win races, I would feel breathless for the short amount of time I could keep up. My heart would beat faster, I would feel uncomfortable, and if they tried to hold a conversation with me, I would struggle. If they matched my pace, they wouldn't feel challenged in any way; in fact, the run would feel more like a slow jog and their heart rate would barely elevate.

If, on the other hand, someone who hadn't run in several years joined me on my early morning run, my pace and the terrain would feel hard to them. This hypothetical person would soon be breathless as we made our way up the first hill and would likely need to walk as we approached the second hill because their lungs would burn and their legs would ache.

All things in life are like this. The person who stands in front of people and lectures for a living will have less of a reaction to public speaking than the person who has never given a talk in front of a group. The person who regularly goes to functions where they don't know anyone and understands how to comfortably strike up conversation with a stranger is going to feel less anxious during social situations than the person who rarely leaves the house. When we expose ourselves to situations—whether physical or emotional—that are appropriately challenging, we adapt so that the anxiety associated with the challenge eventually lessens. If, before we have adapted, the challenge results in a negative experience, our ability to adapt and our reaction to the stimulus changes. If the stimulus is deemed not safe in some way, it's easy to abandon the challenge before adaptation can take place.

In the running example above, if I pushed my pace while running with the fit marathon runners so I was working at a level of 8.5 on a scale from 1 to 10 for more miles than I normally run, that would be a lot of stress on my system. I wouldn't feel great the next day, and it's even possible that I would strain or tweak something because the increased challenge exceeded my physical system's ability to adapt.

What would happen if instead I decided not to worry about keeping up with the marathon runners, but focused on increasing my cadence for 20–30 seconds every two minutes for the duration of my regular run? It would be challenging, but I wouldn't feel battered or injured. In fact, if I did this regularly for a month, I would probably notice I was running a little faster on my regular runs. My body would have an opportunity to adapt to the slight increases in speed. My overall running efficiency and economy would improve because of changes in cellular metabolism and oxygen extraction, and the initial sense of challenge would decrease.

Because aerobic exercise causes changes in heart rate and respiration, it creates an opportunity for those systems to become more finely regulated, especially if aerobic exercise involves changes in resistance or elevation. Each of these changes causes a corresponding change in the cardiovascular system; the amount of cardiovascular response is determined by perception of the activity, past experience, and fitness level.

Let's say you go hiking in the dark, on a trail you don't really know, with extremely trustworthy friends who know the trail well. The goal is to see the sunrise from the top of the hills. Because you can't see in front of you as you hike, you just walk, placing one foot in front of the other, until you reach the peak. When asked how challenging it was, you rate it as moderately hard and say yes, you would absolutely do it again.

Now pretend you are hiking the same trail in daylight. You are well rested, adequately hydrated, and feeling physically prepared. You can see the never-ending hill stretching out in front of you as you begin hiking. It feels hard before you start, and as you near the halfway marker, you feel your heart pounding in your chest and your breath quickening to a point where you don't think you are going to make it to the top. What happened?

Your perception changed, based on your visual input. A South African researcher named Timothy Noakes has spent his career studying the causes of the limitations of human endurance. He doesn't believe it's physiological; our brain, he says, kicks in before our bodies are actually going to give out in order to keep us safe. He calls this the central governor theory, and he posits that it functions to protect the heart from obstruction of blood flow during bouts of exercise nearing maximal capacity (Noakes, 2001).

Why can some people push harder than others? How does seeing the steepness of a hill affect the physical ability to hike up it if all other variables are kept the same? (By the way, I have actually tried the hill experiment a few times while running. I am always surprised by my brain's ability to convince me the hill I ran up in the dark the week before is suddenly monstrous and unconquerable at my normal running pace when the sun is out.) Another way to look at this is that when I am able to see the steep elevation change of the hill I am about to run, it causes me anticipatory anxiety, which increases my heart rate before I even begin running up it. When I can't see the elevation change, I don't experience any anticipatory anxiety and am more relaxed as I make my way up the incline.

The ability to detect changes in heart rate can lead to differences in the ability to respond to a mentally stressful situation as well. In one study, researchers had subjects perform a computerized mental stress task that involved responding rapidly to visual and acoustic stimuli (think flashing lights and dinging sounds). Subjects who could more easily feel their heart rate changing speed as the task became more challenging performed worse and had more negative emotions than subjects who didn't consciously notice their heart rate response (Kindermann & Werner, 2014).

It's not that detecting changes in heart rate is bad, exactly. It's the emotional response that pairs with the realization that "Hey! My heart rate is elevating!" If I looked at the steep hill, felt my heart rate elevate, and said to myself, "I notice my heart rate elevating. That's great. It will provide me with the oxygen I need to get up the hill," my emotional response would be different than if I said to myself, "Crap. That is a big hill. There is no way I am going to make it up that running." In fact, changing my mindset and mental self-talk regarding the stressful task of the hill may even alter how much my heart rate increases (Williams *et al.*, 2017). Changing my emotional response changes my physiological response.

Perhaps the people who are able to push harder are the ones who view an increase in heart rate as a positive thing—as a way to have energy to do what they need to do, and maybe this lack of concern seeps into their response to the stressor, whether it's a physical task or an emotional one. I am not suggesting that you should ask your clients to ignore internal cues; I have known people who have learned to completely ignore feedback from their bodies and then ignored something big. But when the heart is regularly stressed through cardiovascular activity and individuals learn to trust that it will support them and provide adequate blood flow to the muscles so they can rise to the physical or mental challenge, their relationship to an elevated heart rate changes. This, conveniently, is one of the potential reasons cardiovascular exercise seems to have such a powerful impact on anxiety. It exposes people regularly to a physiological response they may currently associate with anxiety or panic without negative consequences. This decrease in sensitivity to physiological sensations can change the individual's perception of their internal strength (Broman-Fulks *et al.*, 2004).

Regularly stressing the heart through aerobic exercise also teaches individuals what normal stress feels like, making it easier to discern when something is abnormal. Interoception becomes more finely tuned and people become more able to read body sensations accurately.

Neurons that fire together, the saying goes, wire together. A neuron is a specialized cell that relays information from one cell to another. Basically, you learn through repetition and consistency. Whether you repeat a behavior, response, motor pattern, or skill often enough for the neurons that cause a specific response to wire together depends on a number of factors, including whether the outcome is deemed favorable and your internal motivation for the behavior.

When you think about something like how regularly stressing the heart through aerobic exercise makes you feel for the rest of the day or what happens when you become more in tune with how the heart rate can increase when you are working hard physically or feeling nervous, you are learning what is normal for you. This type of learning creates connections and makes behavior more or less likely to be repeated, depending on whether it is deemed supportive, injurious, or unhelpful.

Learning

When you were first learning your times tables, more than likely via rote memorization, at some point you learned $9 \times 7 = 63$. The first few times you stared at the numbers 9×7, you probably had to look at the answer and say it to yourself over and over again until every time you looked at the expression 9×7, you knew that the correct answer was 63. The neurons in your brain, through repeated exposure, learned to connect 9, 7, and 63. The meaning you assigned to these three numbers while learning depended largely on the foundation you had previously established or how many other connections your brain had already created between the numbers 9 and 7, and the symbol $\times$. These neural connections enabled you to build on your already established foundation and understand things like multiplication, the complexity of numbers, and quantity.

Building neural connections requires work. If I want to teach someone to do something they perceive as challenging, like a backward roll, I have to first figure out: a) which parts of the backward roll the client can currently do and b) the next attainable part of the backward roll I can teach using coaching skills and environmental context. This is called the zone of proximal development.

In order for the client to learn the next part of the backward roll, it's critical that they feel safe, both in the environment and with my ability to coach the skill. If the client doesn't feel adequately safe, their ability to learn is compromised.

You can't learn what you don't know. Learning requires information, but not too much information. An optimal arousal level is required in order for learning to be successful—if you are falling asleep while learning the backward roll, you probably won't remember much about it the next day. Conversely, if you have just had a triple espresso and feel like the world is moving very, very fast, learning how to navigate your body backward through space with control and ease may not translate to actually learning the different components of the skill (and arguably isn't the best use of your highly caffeinated state).

Optimal arousal is a psychological construct that refers to the optimal level of mental stimulation, where physical performance and learning are maximized. It is closely associated with the state of flow. Flow is a term used in psychology to mean that someone is fully immersed in what they are doing and is a proposed explanation for why people participate in challenging activities, such as learning new skills or writing books (Xie, 2016).

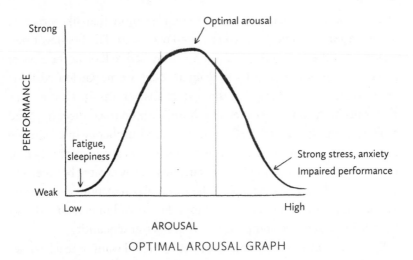

OPTIMAL AROUSAL GRAPH

Learning how to backward roll requires the ability to flex the spine and hips. It also requires a degree of shoulder mobility and the ability to track the trailing foot visually. Before I teach someone how to backward roll, I am going to make sure they have these key skills—if they are missing any of these skills, I will teach the missing skill until it can be translated into a variety of situations. This not only gives the client the necessary information to learn the skill, it also creates a level of security. When you can translate a specific movement, like spinal flexion, into a variety of positions, it will be easier to understand and sense what the body is doing when it is in a precarious and unusual position, like upside down and rotated.

The focused attention required to learn how to do these different skills creates a window of optimal arousal. If I am doing my job well, the student will be engaged, interested, and curious about how these pieces fit together. This will make the teaching of the backward roll more successful.

Brain-Derived Neurotrophic Factor

In order for learning to take place, you need neurons that are able to survive and connect to other neurons. There are specialized molecules that support the survival of neurons, called neurotrophic factors (or cytokines, because sometimes science likes to give things two names). These are soluble (meaning they can dissolve in liquid) proteins (Jain, 2019). There is a special cytokine called brain-derived neurotrophic factor, or BDNF, that allows new neural connections to be made throughout the entirety of your life.

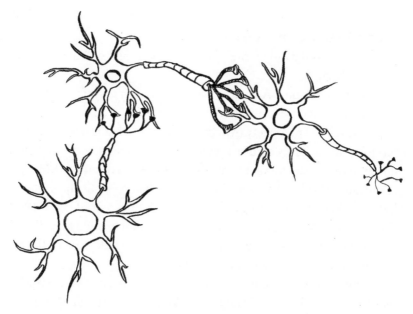

NEURAL CONNECTION

This is excellent news because it means that no matter what happens as you get older, you are still able to learn. The act of learning means you are engaged and curious about yourself and the world around you. What happens if you stop learning or being engaged and curious? It would take a toll on your emotional well-being. Life wouldn't have meaning or purpose. You wouldn't feel like there was a reason to continue moving forward.

The other thing that takes a toll on our ability to learn and, perhaps not surprisingly, the amount of BDNF that is floating around and available for use is chronic long-term stress. Fortunately, we have a non-invasive, built-in defense against the potentially negative effects of long-term stress: aerobic exercise.

So, how much exercise do you need to counteract the effects of chronic stress? Unfortunately, we don't actually know, but scientists are pretty sure it needs to be the cardiovascular type and it should probably be done at least twice a week. In fact, meeting the American College of Sports Medicine (ACSM) minimum recommended requirements of 150 minutes of moderate physical activity a week or 75 minutes of vigorous physical activity a week appears to be enough to protect against chronic stress and improve your ability to learn (Pescatello, 2014).

Aerobic Exercise and Anxiety

"This is all fine and dandy, Jenn," you might be thinking, "but what does the research say?"

A lot, it turns out. A 2018 systematic meta-analysis found that high-intensity exercise is correlated with a decrease in anxiety states and symptoms related to anxiety (Aylett *et al.*, 2018). What is high-intensity exercise, you ask? It is cardiovascular exercise that is performed at a minimum of 60 percent of a person's heart rate maximum (HRM).

You know that breathless feeling you get when you walk up 155 stairs? That's the feeling of working at higher than 60 percent of your HRM. Why 155 stairs? Because it seemed like a good number and I actually did this a couple of weeks ago as a precursor to a hike I like to do—the 155 stairs was a nice way to get warm.

Measuring your current heart rate as a percentage of your HRM is a way to measure how hard you are working. This can also be thought of as your exertion level. If you want to be able to walk a specific route faster or you want to make it up the 155 stairs feeling less breathless, a physiological adaptation has to occur. The kicker is that the only way for these adaptations to happen is if the intensity is high enough that the body responds to the stress.

Think of it this way: if I regularly walk from here to the parking lot at a slow, meandering pace so I can talk to my sister on the phone, my exertion level will be low. I will be working at a low percentage of my HRM. Over time, I might actually get slower because I am not challenging my cardiovascular fitness in any sort of meaningful way.

If instead I walk fast from my workplace to my car, I might feel breathless for the first four weeks, but my body will slowly adapt to the speed and I will feel less breathless while walking at the same speed.

I have a client who usually walks with a good friend. They chat the entire time while walking fast, and the four-mile walk flies by. When she walks with her husband, she walks slower. They chat less and she doesn't feel like she is getting the same workout. If her good friend is out of town for an extended period of time, her walking pace actually decreases and the same four miles of walking feels more challenging. She adapts her physiological response to how social the walk is (we will discuss the benefit of social connections more in Chapter 4).

Maximal oxygen uptake, or VO2 max, is the amount of oxygen the body takes in during inspiration per kilogram of body weight. It's another way to measure exercise intensity (She et al., 2015). If the intensity is regularly too high, the risk of overtraining increases (Nikolaidis et al., 2018). Percentage of VO2 max can be an accurate measure of intensity, but it's pretty unlikely you (or your clients) have access to the expensive lab equipment that measures VO2 max.

Another common way to gauge intensity is by using the percentage of your HRM. There are a few different ways to calculate your HRM, but the thing is, very few people know their HRM.

I spent a bit of time in an exercise science lab during university and I have had both my VO2 max and my HRM tested. My HRM is lower than average for my age but my VO2 max is above average. These numbers mean little, other than that I know not to get too worried about the fact that my heart rate rarely goes over 160, even if I am working quite hard.

Unless you are working with someone with specific goals related to speed and performance, a much easier way to gauge exercise intensity is by using rate of perceived exertion. There are a number of scales that are used to measure exertion, but most people who are working enough to feel a little breathless but still be able to answer a question are more than likely within an acceptable range to elicit physiological (and emotional) adaptations to the exercise stimulus.

There are benefits with working at higher intensities, including, as mentioned above, a higher reduction in anxiety. But one of the biggest issues with high-intensity exercise is the enjoyment factor tends to go down. And when enjoyment goes down, so does the likelihood you will continue to do the exercise on a regular basis (Bottoms *et al.*, 2019). This will be discussed further in subsequent chapters, but the best exercise and intensity for anxiety are those that people will sustain.

So, we know that aerobic exercise may lead to an increase in tolerance to physiological changes and makes learning easier. How else is aerobic exercise beneficial for mental health?

Self-efficacy, which is how you think about your ability to change, is an important aspect of mental health. If my back has been hurting for three months and I think it is going to hurt forever because it is "bad" and I can't change it, I have low self-efficacy. If, on the other hand, I believe I have the power to do something to change my experience of sensation in my low back, my self-efficacy is high.

It turns out that regular aerobic exercise is correlated with higher levels of self-efficacy. The thing about any form of consistent exercise is that over time you will observe changes. The hills get easier, the walks begin to take less time, your lungs burn less. You are changing your physical capacity, which implies you can change in other areas of your life.

When you react to a situation, the reaction is based on your assessment of the sensations within you. These sensations are influenced by your environment, which your body senses through the afferent branch of your PNS. This is also known as exteroception. They are also influenced by how you anticipate your physical reaction will feel. This is called your emotion action tendency (Lowe & Ziemke, 2011). Exercise not only affects our physiology, it also represents a change in behavior, which in turn affects our emotions. Our assessment of sensations changes; so does our ability to perceive what physical responses will feel like.

Cardiovascular activity literally changes the activity in your brain. In order to walk three miles over different types of terrain, the part of your brain that comes up with things like "What if my house burns down and my insurance company decides not to cover for damages and I lose everything?" is less busy because the part of the brain that ensures proper motor output is working to keep you placing one foot in front of the other.

Aerobic exercise is an opportunity for people to reduce anxious rumination. Researchers suggest that exercise poses a distraction for the brain, shifting activity from the frontal and prefrontal cortices to the motor cortices. This shift may result in a change in outlook and perception (Wollseiffen *et al.*, 2018).

I hope by now you are realizing that your brain and the areas of it you regularly use play a large role in how you feel about life. People who are depressed regularly throughout their lives tend to have smaller hippocampal volume than non-depressed individuals (Anand & Dhikav, 2012). The hippocampus is the part of the brain that is important for learning and memory. It's also critical for things like spatial navigating ("How do I get from my house to the grocery store?") and regulation of the ANS (*ibid.*). You learned earlier that aerobic exercise increases the capacity for learning; this is really good for people who struggle with persistent depression.

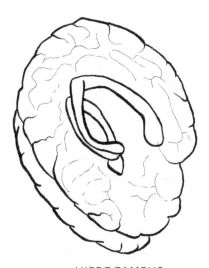

HIPPOCAMPUS

Using your body to get from point A to point B by walking, running, hiking, biking, rollerblading, or paddle boarding is going to increase hippocampus activity because you are navigating space. If you want the brain to be healthy, you need to use all of the parts of the brain. Fortunately, simple aerobic movement taps into some key areas. In fact, research suggests that a regular, moderate-intensity walking program done consistently for a year is enough to increase the volume of the hippocampus (Gujral *et al.*, 2019). Your heart muscle gets stronger and bigger when you exercise, and so does your brain.

People who are clinically depressed also have changes in the parts of the brain associated with interoceptive processing and higher-level executive and motor functions. This means depressed people may not detect when their heart rate is elevated and know why theirs is higher than that of someone who isn't depressed. Depressed individuals may also struggle to perform higher-level motor skills and/or organize the tasks that may be most efficient for something like an obstacle course. Aerobic exercise counteracts these brain changes and actually increases the volume of these areas. The more robust these brain regions are, the higher the likelihood they will protect you against depression later in life.

Meta-analyses have linked depression to a reduction in microstructure integrity of white matter (Jiang *et al.*, 2017). Gray matter is the outermost part of your brain. White matter lies beneath the gray matter and comprises millions of axon bundles. These axon bundles connect the neurons in different brain regions to create functional circuits. The white color comes from the myelin that coats the axons (Fields, 2010). The structural integrity of white matter in healthy older adults who exercise is high; in fact, older and younger individuals who exercise were found to have similar white matter structure, suggesting that exercise may protect the brain against aging. Aerobic exercise interventions are correlated with an increase in structural integrity in white matter for healthy individuals, which may be another reason why aerobic exercise protects against depression during the aging process.

Incorporating Aerobic Exercise: The Laws of Consistency and Gradual Improvement

I have worked with a number of people over the years who come to see me slightly hobbled by their vacations. When I ask what happened, they respond with something like "We walked 5–7 miles a day. I felt fine at the time, but towards the end my back/feet/[insert body part here] really began to hurt."

"How much were you walking before vacation?" I ask.

"Maybe a mile and a half, once a week. But it's just walking. I should've been fine."

What happened? Why did the increase in a normal activity suddenly turn into an uncomfortable experience? If you are over 25 (or maybe 35), whenever you increase your physical activity without giving your system a chance to adapt to the new stress, your system rebels. Even though many don't consider walking exercise, it is still a repetitive load throughout the entire body. You wouldn't go from doing no push-ups to 15 push-ups every day for a week without expecting soreness and discomfort; going from occasional walking to daily walking for hours at a time is the same. Repetitive load is repetitive load, and your body needs an opportunity to adapt through incremental doses.

When you are giving guidance to someone who is just beginning an exercise program or who wants to participate in an activity outside of their normal routine, there are a few rules to adhere to in order to ensure the person is successful. When someone has been inactive or sedentary for a long period of time, both their perception of what they "should" be able to do and your interpretation of what is adequate to make an impact on their emotional state may need to be adjusted. The ACSM recommends 30 minutes of moderate aerobic activity five times a week. Based on your and your client's previous experience, that may sound like either a lot or very little. Let's approach this from both scenarios.

"I used to be really fit. Thirty minutes isn't enough." Occasionally, you may be working with someone who was an athlete in their younger years but for one reason or another has been inactive for a long stretch of time. This person tends to have a "go big or go home" attitude and may be perplexed by the idea of doing less than an hour of physical activity a day in their quest to "get back in shape." But—and this is a big but—this individual hasn't been active for years, and while they may build a foundation faster than someone who hasn't ever been active, they still need to build a foundation. This idea will show up repeatedly throughout the rest of the book: when you ask someone prone to anxiety to perform more than their tissues or nervous system is prepared to handle, negative sensation increases, causing discomfort and decreasing the likelihood of consistency.

On the other end of the spectrum is the client struggling with kinesiophobia, or fear of movement. This client is afraid of injuring themselves and is concerned exercise will make all of their musculo-skeletal conditions worse. With these individuals, you can begin with an even smaller dose of exercise. You could suggest a five-minute walk twice a day. While this might not seem like much, in the beginning it's not about the quantity of the exercise; rather, it's about performing the exercise consistently—creating a habit that can be maintained for the rest of the person's life.

Now that you understand the neural mechanisms behind aerobic exercise and the basic psychology involved in why aerobic exercise works in individuals struggling with anxiety, Chapter 3 will explore the mental health benefits of another facet of exercise: strength.

References

Anand K.S., & Dhikav V. (2012). Hippocampus in health and disease: An overview. Annals of Indian Academy of Neurology, 15(4), 239-246.

Aylett E., Small N., & Bower P. (2018). Exercise in the treatment of clinical anxiety in general practice: A systematic review and meta-analysis. BMC Health Services Research, 18, 559.

Bottoms L., Leighton D., Carpenter R., Anderson S., et al. (2019). Affective and enjoyment responses to 12 weeks of high intensity interval training and moderate continuous training in adults with Crohn's disease. PLOS ONE, 14(9), 1-13.

Broman-Fulks J.J., Berman M.E., Rabian B.A., & Webster M.J. (2004). Effects of aerobic exercise on anxiety sensitivity. Behavior Research and Therapy, 42(2), 125-136.

Cornelissen V.A., Verheyden B., Aubert A.E., & Fagard R.H. (2010). Effects of aerobic training intensity on resting, exercise and post exercise blood pressure, heart rate and heart-rate variability. Journal of Human Hypertension, 24(3), 175-182.

Fields R.D. (2010). Neuroscience. Change in the brain's white matter. Science, 330(6005), 768-769.

Garfinkle S.N., Manassei M.F., Hamilton-Fletcher G., In den Bosch Y., Critchley H.D., & Engels M. (2016). Interoceptive dimensions across cardiac and respiratory axes. Philosophical Transactions of the Royal Society of London Series B Biological Sciences, 371(1708), 1-10.

Gujral S., Aaizenstein H., Reynolds III C.F., Butters M.A., & Erickson K.I. (2019). Exercise effects on depression: Possible neural mechanisms. General Hospital Psychiatry, 49, 2-10.

Huang J., Uke C., Sander S., Jawinski J., Hegeri U, & Hensch T. (2018). Impact of brain arousal and time-on-task on autonomic nervous system activity in the wake-sleep transition. BMC Neuroscience 19, 18.

Jain K.K. (2019). Neurotrophic factors. Neuropharmacology & Neurotherapeutics: Medlink. Accessed on November 10, 2022 at www.medlink.com/articles/neurotrophic-factors.

Jiang J., Zhao Y-J., Hu X-Y., Du M-Y., et al. (2017). Microstructural brain abnormalities in medication-free patients with major depressive disorder: A systematic review and meta-analysis of diffusion tensor imaging. Journal of Psychiatry & Neuroscience, 42(3), 150-163.

Kindermann N.K., & Werner N.S. (2014). The impact of cardiac perception on emotion experience and cognitive performance under mental stress. Journal of Behavioral Medicine, 37(6), 1145-1154.

Laforgia J., Withers R.T., & Gore C.J. (2006). Effects of exercise intensity and duration on the excess post-exercise oxygen consumption. Journal of Sports Sciences, 24(12), 1247-1264.

Lofrese J.J., & Lappin S.L. (2019). Physiology, residual volume. In: Statpearls [Internet]. Treasure Island, FL: Statpearls Publishing.

Lowe R., & Ziemke T. (2011). The feeling of action tendencies: On the emotional regulation of goal-directed behavior. Frontiers in Psychology, 2, 346.

Nikolaidis P.T., Rosemann T., & Knechtle B. (2018). Age-predicted maximal heart rate in recreational marathon runners: A cross-sectional study on Fox's and Tanaka's equations. Frontiers in Physiology, 9, 226.

Noakes T.D. (2001). Evidence that a central governor regulates exercise performance during acute hypoxia and hyperoxia. Journal of Experimental Biology, 204(18), 3225-3234.

Pescatello L.S. (2014). ACSM's Guidelines for Exercise Testing and Prescription. 9th edition. Philadelphia, PA: Wolters Kluwer/Lippincott Williams & Wilkins Health.

Price C.J., & Hooven C. (2018). Interoceptive awareness skills for emotion regulation: Theory and approach of mindful awareness in body-oriented therapy (MABT). Frontiers in Psychology, 9, 798.

Sasaki K., & Maruyama R. (2014). Consciously controlled breathing decreases the high-frequency component of heart rate variability by inhibiting cardiac parasympathetic nerve activity. Tohoku Journal of Experimental Medicine, 233(3), 155-163.

She J., Nakamura H., Makino K., Ohyama Y., & Hashimoto H. (2015). Selection of suitable maximum-heart-rate formulas for use with Karvonen formulas to calculate exercise intensity. International Journal of Automation and Computing, 12(1), 62-69.

West B.J., & Turalska M. (2019). Hypothetical control of heart rate variability. Frontiers in Physiology, 10, 1078.

Williams S.E., Veldhuijzen van Zanten J.J.C.S., Trotman G.P., Quinton M.L., & Ginty A.T. (2017). Challenge and threat imagery manipulates heart rate and anxiety response to stress. International Journal of Psychophysiology, 117, 111-118.

Wollseiffen P., Vogt T., Struder H.K., & Schneider S. (2018). Distraction versus intensity: The importance of exercise classes for cognitive performance in school. Medical Principles and Practice: International Journal of the Kuwait University, Health Science Centre, 27(1), 61-65.

Xie P.F. (2016). Optimal Arousal. In: Jafari J., & Xiao H. (eds) Encyclopedia of Tourism. Cham: Springer.

Your Lungs and Exercise (2016). Breathe, 12(1), 97-100.

CHAPTER 3

The Power of Strength

I have a client who is in the early stages of dementia. She has always been anxious, but she doesn't associate many of her physical ailments with her anxiety. Whenever she and her husband are going on a big trip, she breaks out in hives. As soon as she arrives at her destination, the hives disappear.

During the pandemic, she and her husband didn't travel and she was consistent with her strength-training routine, seeing me twice a week and using her weighted balls at home periodically in between sessions.

At her six-month follow-up appointment with her neurologist, he told her the dementia symptoms hadn't increased; in fact, if anything, they were a little bit better. She is noticeably calmer now, and her anxious tics I used to notice during our sessions have almost entirely disappeared. Building strength has made her more mentally strong.

When someone lacks a feeling of physical strength, their proprioception is altered. Proprioception is a sense, like smell or vision, that tells you things like where your right arm is located while you read this, how your right foot feels against the floor, how much force you need to turn the page, and how fast your hand needs to move to turn the page (Ager et al., 2019). It is the unconscious knowledge of how to accomplish a movement task based on the range of motion available.

When you can't easily feel your body's position in space, your emotional state might be affected. Or perhaps it's the other way around. Research suggests that when people feel fear or anxiety, postural stability is impaired (Davis et al., 2011). This may cause you to feel afraid of falling or to lack confidence on unstable surfaces or terrain. Whether or not you feel your environment poses a threat plays an important role in spatial perception, postural control, and locomotion; it stands to reason, then, that someone prone to feelings of anxiety will have an altered sense of their body and how they maneuver through the world (Staab *et al.*, 2013).

TRY THIS: When you think of feeling anxious, what words come to mind? Don't judge them, simply jot them down in the notes on your phone or on a notepad.

Now look over your list. Read the first word out loud and pause. How does it make your body feel?

Read the rest of the words on your list out loud, pausing after each one so you have time to register the internal feeling states that accompany them.

Now try the same exercise, but instead of thinking of feeling anxious, think of feeling depressed or blue. How do those words make your body feel?

Critical analysis is generally a (mostly) top-down process (see Chapter 1 for more on top-down and bottom-up processing). When you look at someone and try and assess their movement through critical thinking, you are using top-down processing.

Bottom-up processing is based on the sensations that arise in the body—the interoceptive cues that constantly inform our thinking state. The ability to notice these interoceptive cues and not judge them is another way to experience emotion. Instead of telling a client how they should feel in a specific exercise, asking them what they are experiencing gives them an opportunity to utilize bottom-up processing during the task.

Curiously, when you ask someone who isn't accustomed to using bottom-up processing what they are experiencing, they may struggle to find the right words to describe their experience. I see this regularly—in fact, some of my long-time clients roll their eyes when I ask and tell me, "I don't know what I'm feeling. I'll let you know tomorrow."

Focusing is a process developed by Eugene Gendlin, a psychologist, that teaches people how to pay attention to vague physical impressions until they become less vague and more meaningful (Shalev, 2018). Feelings around words such as "anxiety" or "depression" often lead to other words that we experience on a somatic or visceral level.

Let's pretend you are afraid of spiders. If you were to see an eight-legged object that resembled a spider your SNS would kick in, activating your fear response by spiking your blood pressure and heart rate, and making you breathe faster. Later, if you found out it was actually a toy spider, you would laugh but you might still feel uneasy—the visual representation of a spider is enough to trigger fear.

This is an example of low stress tolerance—reacting to something that looks like it might be stressful as if it were stressful even if it really isn't. Low stress tolerance is characterized by the desire for predictability, a preference for order and structure, and a low tolerance for ambiguity (Iannello *et al.*, 2017). When emotions are undifferentiated and everything outside of a very controlled set of circumstances is considered stressful, it becomes difficult to relax. Emotional and physical health is affected because of the perpetual state of heightened SNS activity.

I occasionally teach yoga to high-ranking military officers. One of the questions they inevitably ask while they are getting out the mats is "How should we set up the room?"

"However you want," I respond.

There is a pause as everyone looks at each other. They adhere to order and predictability when it's available; having someone tell them they can set their things wherever they want isn't orderly or predictable.

Eventually, they line the yoga mats up in a very logical way. The emphasis the military places on order and predictability whenever possible makes sense. When you spend your days in situations that are at times ambiguous and chaotic, you find structure in other places in order to maintain some sort of balance. If you put so much emphasis on structure that you forget to be adaptable and flexible, it puts a strain on relationships, creates somatic health issues, and affects your mood. There is a happy medium in there somewhere; tapping into bottom-up processing can help you find it.

In traditional exercise settings, the environment is predictable. There are mats and blocks if you are in a yoga studio, reformers and mats if you are in a Pilates studio, and rubber flooring and weights if you are in a gym. Often, the exercises go in a specific order and the experience is put together with a sense of structure. This creates a low-stress environment, which is good for learning and is great for people with a low stress tolerance but can also feed into a more rigid mindset regarding movement and fitness. I am not suggesting that everyone should create chaotic client environments, because that's not conducive for learning and isn't a good environment for the person teaching. But, as you will see in Chapter 6, if you occasionally create a less predictable order or structure, you will actually facilitate more client autonomy and focus. This translates to both the exercises the client is performing and the client's ability to discern feeling.

Interoception and Its Role in Movement

Interoception, the internal sense of the body, includes feelings related to muscular tightness and instability. Like the other senses, interoception is influenced by emotional states. Breathing, for instance, can be altered by heightened anxiety, and altering breathing patterns can alter levels of arousal (Paulus, 2013). When breathing patterns change, posture also changes, which affects proprioception.

Proprioception is an important element of motor control and coordination; when proprioception is altered because of how someone is feeling emotionally, it impacts control of muscle tone and postural reflexes (Aman *et al.*, 2015). One way to alter muscle tone is through applied force, either as an external load or through isometric contraction. The effects of force on the senses are twofold: the sensation of muscular work is an interoceptive sense and the change in muscle tone changes proprioception.

"I can't feel my body"

Sometimes I ask clients to feel how they are moving their arms/legs/spine/shoulder blades/feet/elbows/etc. Sometimes people know exactly what I'm talking about and can make a mental connection with that specific body part, and sometimes they can't.

If you can't feel a specific body part and its position, all of the words in the world won't change how you are doing a movement. You can't change what you can't feel. Improving proprioception and its conscious component, kinesthetic awareness, is what enables you to move a specific area differently.

I have a client who used to perform leg exercises by swinging her right hip out to the right. She couldn't feel herself doing it, so I used movements rather than words to demonstrate her normal strategy.

By using things like a wall, her hand, or a strap, she began to have a more clear image of the right half of the pelvis and how it moved.

Once she began to feel the location of her right hip and how its position affected what she felt in her leg, torso, and shoulder, she began to play with her position throughout the week. She would notice when her right hip swayed out and would try alternative strategies.

Over time, she found herself thinking about it less, but she could easily draw her attention there if asked. The back pain across her right low back disappeared and she felt more willing to try new exercises and move in different ways.

Before moving on, it's worthwhile to note that interoceptive senses can have varying degrees of focus and accuracy. If you asked ten executives how they were feeling 30 minutes before lunch some may answer, "Hungry," others may answer, "I am a bit shaky and light-headed, and I feel like my blood pressure is dipping lower than it should," and a third group may answer, "Just fine. Why do you ask?"

The executives who answer, "Hungry" are demonstrating interoceptive accuracy. They are able to feel and accurately interpret their internal bodily senses and probably have a good handle on what different physical sensations mean and represent.

The executives who give the long answer by overanalyzing their blood sugar levels are demonstrating an increased attentional focus on their physical states. This type of interoceptive body awareness isn't necessarily bad if it isn't reflective of the way a person regularly thinks about what's happening physiologically. If, on the other hand, it is the way they normally experience and analyze their body sensations, it could potentially be unhealthy and maladaptive. Increased attentional focus on the physical state is associated with things like anxiety, hypervigilance, and tendencies towards hypochondria.

The executives who didn't check in with their internal cues at all are demonstrating low interoceptive awareness (Mehling *et al.*, 2018). They aren't in tune with their internal physical states, and it would be challenging for this hypothetical group to connect their hunger with, for example, their short, slightly angry answer to an employee's question five minutes later.

You are probably noticing that the ability to interpret the senses exists across a scale. If you are taking a holistic approach towards movement, exercise, and mental health, figuring out the optimal position on the scale for the person in front of you will go a long way towards them creating a more balanced way of existing in the world. The desk worker who doesn't view exercise as enjoyable doesn't need the same amount of kinesthetic awareness as the recreational dancer, just like the United States Navy captain probably doesn't need as much interoceptive accuracy as the mind/body therapist. The optimization of experience is different for everyone. My goal is always to meet people where they are, not where I think they should be.

Because interoception is considered a foundation for both physiological and psychological experience, it's important for the practitioner to recognize when the client is hyper-focused on interoceptive instructions or when the client lacks interoceptive awareness and/or isn't sensitive to interoceptive-based direction (Duquette, 2017). The exercises and instructions used in a movement session should reflect the client's needs. Let's consider two examples.

Amy is a thoughtful, intelligent person who experiences a lot of sensation throughout her torso and arms. She can readily describe muscular sensations, which she interprets as pain, and she is afraid of exercising because she is worried she is going to make the sensations she experiences worse. Should interoceptive instruction (words that ask the client to reflect on their internal experience) be used? Probably not at first. Because Amy is demonstrating heightened interoceptive awareness, which is correlated with trait anxiety, she will benefit from a movement-based program that doesn't emphasize internal sensations initially (Pollatos *et al.*, 2007). Kinesiophobia, or fear of movement, isn't uncommon in people who have chronic pain. If Amy thinks movements are going to cause more pain, there is a pretty good chance she is going to brace or guard before she even starts the movement. Muscle guarding can include things like hesitating to perform a movement, stiffening, and/or bracing unnecessarily (Olugbade *et al.*, 2019).

Imagine what it would feel like if you braced as though you were going to deadlift 300 pounds every time you bent over to pick up a napkin from the floor. It sounds exhausting. The thought of moving in a specific way can cause this tensing, or guarding, prior to the movement and is correlated with anxiety (*ibid.*). In fact, a study concluded that addressing how people with chronic pain move may increase their physical activity more than focusing on how much they move (*ibid.*).

If Amy anticipates lifting a weight will hurt her back, it will hurt her back. Empowering Amy through task-based movement skills is an entryway to improving her interoceptive accuracy without drawing her attention to her interoceptive state. We will discuss this further in Chapter 7.

Dan is an engineer who thinks linearly and doesn't spend much time reflecting on how he is feeling internally. Recently, he experienced a bout of persistent back pain when he bent over to pick up a golf ball. He is surprised it hasn't gone away, despite the fact that he is still lifting weights and uses the cardio machines at the gym regularly. When you observe Dan lifting weights, it is clear he moves between exercises quickly, not focusing on how he executes the movements. Should interoceptive instruction be used? Yes. Dan will benefit from slowing down, focusing on the movements, and reflecting on what he is experiencing. Improving his interoceptive awareness may even segue into him being able to more accurately gauge how he feels emotionally and make him feel more in tune with the present moment (Seth *et al.*, 2011). More ideas for how to design movement interventions for clients like Dan will be discussed in Chapter 10.

Strength-based tasks can be instructed and used in a multitude of ways. Emphasizing feeling can enhance the connection between the mind and the body, in addition to improving proprioception and interoception.

Emphasizing completion of a specific task, like setting a weighted object down on tables of different heights, can improve self-confidence ("I can do it!") and feelings of resilience. These are the types of activities that would really benefit Amy. Taking the time to talk to people and understand how they process experiences related to movement can assist you in choosing the appropriate instruction and task for the person with whom you are working.

> **A Quick Note about the Purposeful Omission of the Word "Cue"**
>
> You may notice I am choosing the word "instruction" rather than the word "cue" when I describe different teaching or coaching scenarios. "Cue" is defined by dictionary.com (2022) as a signal to a performer to begin a specific action, a feature, such as the expression on a person's face, that provides a clue to an action, a stimulus, or a sensory signal that identifies experiences or responses. Our words when we instruct are (usually) not actually cues; they are suggestions to try something a different way, not a stimulus or prompt to begin a certain action. In an effort to be clear, the word "instruction" will be used.

The Default Mode Network and Focused Attention

When you are driving to work thinking about what you are going to do later in the week, you are using your default mode network, the part of your brain that is activated when your mind is wandering.

When you are staring intently at the pieces of a puzzle trying to figure out how to connect the edges, you are using your executive control network. This is the part of your brain that is activated when your attention is focused on something external. Or internal: it turns out that directing attention to something specific related to you or to something in the environment can shift brain activation patterns. There is a relationship between having the ability to easily switch from letting your mind wander to focusing your attention on something and anxiety: people who can switch back and forth between these two states tend to have lower levels of anxiety compared to people who struggle with switching modes (Tao *et al.*, 2015).

Since both internally focused attention and externally focused attention appear to decrease activity in the default mode network, this opens up possibilities for your work with clients (Scheibner *et al.*, 2017). It means there isn't a "right" choice when it comes to helping someone become more fluid in their ability to move from a focused to a less focused state. Attentional instruction can be based on the individual.

Before moving on, take a moment to reflect on the everyday movement of getting out of a chair. How many ways can you direct attention or instruct the movement from an internal perspective? How many ways can you direct attention or instruct the movement from an external perspective?

The more options you have for teaching and instructing basic movements, the more likely you are to be able to find a way to focus a client's attention. If the client struggles with focused attention, developing this skill in a movement setting will make their thinking more flexible and adaptable.

Strength and Anxiety

Building strength through movement can improve interoceptive accuracy, improve stress tolerance, increase feelings of resilience, and improve attention.

People who have been diagnosed with anxiety and people who

experience anxiety symptoms but haven't been diagnosed with a mental illness have fewer symptoms related to anxiety when they adopt a strength-based program (Gordon *et al.*, 2017). Strength training makes you feel more capable and less breakable. It requires focus to lift something heavy, and it calibrates how you gauge what's happening internally. Just like learning that running up a hill makes your heart rate increase significantly but nothing bad happens, the physical sense of work that corresponds with using your body to navigate a heavy weight dissipates when you set the weight down. The contrast between work and rest makes it easier to find balance.

This correlation probably doesn't come as much of a surprise. Research clearly shows a link, and anyone who has spent time developing the skill of getting stronger in a progressive, thoughtful way will tell you that something shifts mentally when you know you have the ability to move the 50-pound bag of dog food across the room or you can hold your grandchild without experiencing back pain (Gordon *et al.*, 2017). A meta-analysis of 16 articles involved 922 subjects and concluded that resistance training improved anxiety symptoms among both healthy subjects and those with a physical or mental illness (*ibid.*).

Remember earlier when you wrote down words related to anxiety? Were any of your words related to not feeling grounded, or overthinking, or maybe some combination of both? A lack of physical strength is often accompanied by feeling disconnected from the physical self. Sensation in the form of muscular work re-establishes a connection between the mind and the body. It reminds us on a cognitive level that "Oh yeah. I have a body and I can do things with it that make me feel strong."

Anxiety is correlated with a number of physical conditions, including:

- chronic pain (Mills *et al.*, 2019)
- fatigue (Vassend *et al.*, 2018)
- joint hypermobility syndrome (Bulbena-Cabre & Bulbena, 2018)
- migraines (Peres *et al.*, 2017).

All of these conditions make the idea of exercise unappealing. No one wants to move when they hurt, are tired, or feel physically unstable, or when their head is causing feelings associated with nausea, dizziness, or pain. The conundrum lies in the fact that exercise, specifically resistance training, can positively impact most of these conditions through a reduction in symptom severity.

Strength Training and Chronic Low Back Pain

I have a client who is convinced bending over to pick something up is going to injure his back. He squats down to lift heavy objects and I have to employ tricky instructions to get him to bend over and reach.

This client has chronic low back that has plagued him for most of his life. He is pretty sure exercise is potentially harmful, and he will occasionally look over at what other trainers are doing and tell me, "I can't do that. That would hurt my back." Like Amy, he has a lot of fear around specific movements and a heightened sense of interoception.

This client has also struggled with both depression and anxiety over the years. He goes through periods where he sees me regularly and periods where he doesn't see me at all. When he sees me regularly, he feels better—stronger, more capable, and more confident. When he doesn't see me, his spouse tells me he is less optimistic, less cheerful, and has more pain.

Chronic pain is a serious condition, one that affects 20.4 percent of adults in the United States each year (Dahlhamer *et al.*, 2018). It's more prevalent in older adults and women, and is correlated with depression and anxiety (Vadivelu *et al.*, 2017; Cimpean & David, 2019).

The fear of pain or pain intensification is also frequently seen in people who experience chronic pain. Have you ever sprained your ankle? If so, you probably remember the tentative first step you took in the morning as you tested out how it was feeling.

You might also remember the moment when you "knew" you could put all of your weight on it without worrying how it would feel, because the injury was healing. If you had continued to worry about how it would feel when you put weight on it, you would have been fearful of the possible pain. This type of fear can create a self-fulfilling loop—the anticipatory muscle tensing that occurs before you actually put weight into your ankle makes your ankle hurt more. Your brain goes, "Aha! I knew it was going to hurt," and the cycle continues. Remember earlier when I talked about muscle guarding? If you are afraid your ankle will hurt, you will move in a way that would make an observer say, "Oh wow. That person's ankle must really hurt," even if the tissue is fully healed.

This happens frequently in people with chronic low back pain. Because they are worried certain movements are going to hurt, they move their low backs less.

Resistance training reduces fear related to movement, builds confidence, and instills a sense of resilience. As you will see later in the chapter, there are different ways to introduce strength-based tasks to people with chronic pain and anxiety around movement that feel safe and less intimidating, which is important for building confidence and creating consistency.

Joint Hypermobility Syndrome and Pain

A client began seeing me for chronic pelvic pain. When I asked more about her history, she told me she had experienced several ankle sprains, was a former dancer, and was pretty sure she knew which muscles were working and which weren't. As she began moving, it became obvious that not only was she hypermobile, she also had a lot of fear associated with moving "right."

Joint hypermobility syndrome (JHS) is a genetic connective tissue disorder that results in excessive range of motion at multiple joints and chronic musculoskeletal pain. It affects approximately 3 percent of the population and is related to feelings of anxiety and panic (Kumar & Lenert, 2017; Eccles *et al.*, 2012).

Fortunately, increasing strength makes joints feel more stable and decreases pain in people with JHS. Research suggests that a basic strength-training program of three to five exercises is enough to improve neuromuscular control and improve general strength (Salles *et al.*, 2015).

Later on in the chapter, we will examine ways to introduce strength training to more sensitive clients, such as those struggling with chronic musculoskeletal pain as a result of JHS. For now, know that feeling able to extend the arm without shoulder dislocation can impact how confident and strong someone feels during their day-to-day activities.

Migraines and Strength Training

I have a client who has a very high-stress job and is prone to migraine headaches. She used to cancel when she felt a migraine coming on, concerned that working out would make her migraine worse.

One day she came in, despite the signs that a migraine was coming. I had her work around it, using basic strength exercises and avoiding changes in head position and balance.

At the end of the session, I cautiously asked her how she felt. "Much better," she said, surprised.

Since then, when she feels a migraine coming on, she no longer cancels. We do what we can, and I ask her for feedback if I'm unsure whether a movement is appropriate. Our sessions have never made a migraine feel worse—only better.

Migraines are correlated with anxiety, and strength training reduces symptoms related to anxiety. It makes sense that participating in activities that reduce feelings related to anxiety might decrease the severity of the migraine. This hypothesis is supported by research: having some form of physical practice (either aerobic or strength training) is correlated with a reduction in physical disability of migraine headaches (Domingues *et al.*, 2011). Just like people with chronic pain and anxiety are likely to be fearful of the pain intensifying, women who suffer from migraines and anxiety are more likely to avoid vigorous, moderate-intensity physical activity because of concern that it will trigger a migraine (Farris *et al.*, 2019).

It is important to be sensitive to people's beliefs when you are working with them in the context of introducing physical activity of any kind into their lives. Think back to earlier when I asked you to think about the everyday movement of getting out of a chair. What are the most fundamental principles needed to get out of a chair? And could you regress it even further from there? Examples will be discussed in Chapter 8, but for now, be aware that understanding how to make an aspect of a movement in some way accessible to a client who is worried or concerned about the act of moving will make them feel successful. I am very purposeful in my exercise selection when my client has migraine symptoms. We don't dwell on the symptoms, but she knows that if she feels worse at any time, she can let me know and I will reroute. Conversely, I try to offer appropriate physical challenges and give her something semi-interesting to focus on, taking the attention temporarily away from the discomfort in her head.

Finally, it's important to remember that chronic low back pain, JHS, and migraines are all associated with feelings of fatigue. Pain makes you tired; so does anxiety. Fortunately, resistance training has a positive effect on chronic fatigue. Plus, it has additional benefits, like improving balance and strength (Guillamo *et al.*, 2016). When your balance and strength improve, efficiency during functional activities improves. When efficiency is improved, less energy is expended overall, so the work it takes to build strength is counterbalanced by the decrease in energy required by activities of daily living.

Forms of Strength Training

Load can be applied to skeletal muscle in a variety of ways. When you walk, a series of contractions occurs to overcome gravity and slow down the impact incurred as the foot strikes the ground. Below is a brief overview of some of the more commonly utilized forms of contraction.

Concentric contractions occur when the muscle is shortening while overcoming an external force.

TRY THIS: Come into a seated position on a chair with your feet flat on the floor and your arms reaching out in front of you. Start pressing the feet firmly into the ground. Keep pressing the feet into the ground as you push the ground away from you and stand up. What just happened?

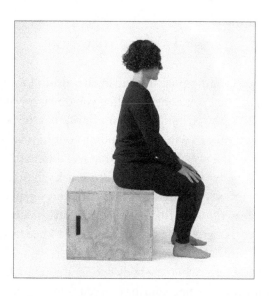

The quadriceps muscles in the front of the thighs shortened to extend the knee and move the torso away from the ground, making this movement a concentric contraction for the quadriceps muscles (there are many other things going on in the hip and torso but let's just focus on the quadriceps muscle group for now). In this case, gravity is the external resistance; it is trying to pull you down, and you resist gravity by moving away from it.

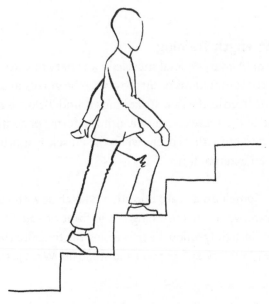

CONCENTRIC CONTRACTION

Now, from the standing position, push the ground away from you strongly. Imagine that someone is pulling you down towards your seat and you are resisting by pushing the ground away, but the person pulling you down is beginning to win, slowly pulling your hips back to the seat until you sit all of the way down. Does that feel different?

More than likely, that felt like more work, though, curiously, eccentric contractions require less muscular energy expenditure than concentric contractions. In this example, the quadriceps muscles are lengthening, working to resist gravity, while the knee flexes. A recent definition of eccentric contractions by researchers says that they dissipate mechanical energy while the body decelerates (Franchi *et al.*, 2017). Eccentric contractions happen during everyday movement to slow down the gravitational pull, like when you walk down stairs or lean over to get something from the bottom shelf of the refrigerator (*ibid.*). I think of eccentric contractions as the ability to dance with gravity—if the dance is in some way synchronous, you have an element of control (and who doesn't like having an element of control?).

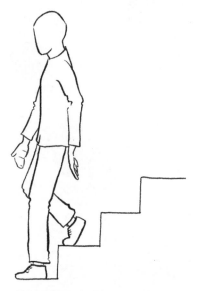

ECCENTRIC CONTRACTION

Bend your elbow as strongly as you can, making your biceps muscle pop. Hold that position for a count of five and then relax. Congratulations! You just performed an isometric contraction.

Isometric contractions are contractions that aren't associated with any actual movement. Though there is no displacement in the joint, there is displacement within the muscle itself at a microscopic level (Buchanan *et al.*, 2004). Isometric contractions act as a pain reliever and are linked to an immediate decrease in painful sensations for people struggling with tendinopathy (Rio *et al.*, 2017). You can perform isometric contractions an infinite number of ways, and these types of contractions can be taught using attention that is focused internally or externally.

Isotonic contractions are defined as the movement of load at constant tension through a defined arc of motion (Ombregt, 2013). Isotonic contractions comprise both concentric and eccentric contractions (the muscle shortens and lengthens while tension is kept constant) and are frequently used in rehabilitative settings (Marri & Swaminathan, 2016).

TRY THIS: Come into a seated position on a chair with your feet flat on the ground and fairly close to the chair. Begin pressing the feet strongly into the ground, as though you are about to stand up, but stay seated. Do you feel your legs working?

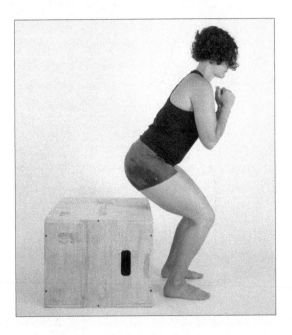

Now press your feet so hard into the floor that your hips come one inch off the chair. Hold that position for three breaths. Lower your hips back down to the chair and relax.

These are examples of isometric contractions at slightly different angles. Despite the fact that the hips are supported in the first version, the mere act of pressing the feet into the ground strongly generates work through the musculature of the thigh. This could be instructed a variety of ways, focusing the contraction in different places throughout the legs. We will discuss this in further detail in a moment when we look at directing attention to different people.

Remain seated on the chair, but imagine that a friend has placed their hands on your shoulders and is gently pressing you down. Begin pressing through your feet to stand up, while resisting the downward push of your friend, who is pushing down consistently the entire time.

When you get to the standing position, imagine that your friend is now pushing down with more force than you can resist, even though you are trying not to let them. Keep resisting while you slowly lower back down to the seated position, with your friend pushing you down using the same amount of force the entire time.

This is an example of an isotonic contraction during a squat-type exercise. Hopefully, all of the variations of muscular contractions felt slightly different and enabled you to tap into different muscular sensations.

Directing Attention for Different People

The contractions above were depicted using words that focused the attention externally. The attention was focused outside the body rather than on the body and how it was performing the action. If, during the concentric contraction exercise, I had asked you to press the feet into the ground, feel the muscular contraction in the quadriceps, and use those muscles to stand up, it would have been an internally focused direction. Or if, during the isometric contraction, I had asked you to press your feet into the ground, feel the muscular work in the front of the thighs, and dial up the work to create more tension in the front of the legs, it would have required an internal focus of attention. Is one better than the other? Not necessarily. At the risk of sounding like a broken record, the type of instructions or descriptions you use depends on the person's relationship with interoception and their ability to focus on bodily sensations.

There is some research suggesting that when you focus on a movement task or external component of a movement, the movement occurs more automatically (Ille *et al.*, 2013). This automatic movement process can be disrupted when you focus on the internal aspects of a movement.

TRY THIS: Set six objects on the floor in a loose line. Walk along the line of objects, reaching down to touch each object as you walk.

Now stand alongside the line of objects with your right foot forward and your left foot behind. Bend both knees so you can touch the first object. Step the left foot forward so your right foot is behind. Bend both knees so you can touch the next object. Repeat until you touch all of the objects.

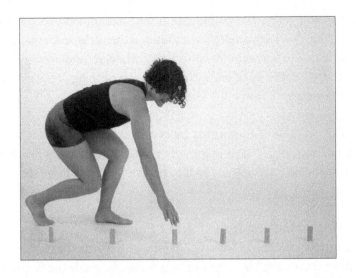

Did these two conditions feel different? Probably. During the second variation, you thought about a specific internal action: bending the knees. This changes how you coordinate all of your body parts to achieve the goal of touching the object. In the first variation, you probably didn't think about bending your knees at all (and the chances are pretty good that you still bent them, unless you are blessed with great hip flexibility and can reach the floor easily without bending your knees).

And this is the thing about different types of directions—if someone is like Amy, then simply moving and not thinking about what they are doing it is going to be hugely beneficial. Having a goal that: a) involves coordinating a variety of joints and b) doesn't cause pain changes the narrative from "Bending over might hurt" to "I can successfully touch objects on the floor while walking."

On the other end of the spectrum is the person who always performs movements in exactly the same way and doesn't even realize that they have a choice. Asking that person to do the movement in a specific way, such as by bending the knees, breaks the automatic process. This is good! Sometimes we need automatic. Sometimes we need conscious awareness. The ability to utilize both internally and externally focused attention benefits both the person instructing and the person receiving the instruction.

The Role of Dopamine in Motor Learning

Dopamine is a neurotransmitter that plays a critical role in reward and movement regulation (Olguin *et al.*, 2015). You know that warm fuzzy feeling you experience when you accomplish something that's challenging? That's dopamine being released, letting your brain know that what you did was worth repeating. It's the reason people do things that seem crazy, like climb Yosemite's Half Dome without ropes or try to run a marathon in under two hours. It's also the reason telling someone, "Thank you. You did great today," can have a profound impact on their mood. We are wired to seek rewarding experiences on a cortical level.

When you are learning a new motor skill, dopamine is released when the new motor memory is encoded. The encoding of new motor memories is what lets you do the same movement pattern again and achieve a similar result (Kawashima *et al.*, 2012). Not only does the feel-good jolt of dopamine make you more likely to repeat the action because your chances of success have gone up, it also increases motivation.

"Motor noise" is a term used to describe variance in motor control. If you stood up and did 100 lunges right now, they wouldn't all be exactly the same. Some may even be less smooth or more awkward than normal. That's motor noise.

Motor noise is a normal part of motor learning. You need a moment (or two) when you are first learning how to do something new to figure out: a) the goal behind the movement and b) how to coordinate your body parts so you can successfully accomplish the goal. Researchers suggest that increased motivation may decrease motor noise, allowing you to more accurately perform the movement (Manohar *et al.*, 2015).

When you teach a client how to do something new or complex, giving them space to try a few times and figure out the basic coordination can be an invaluable part of the learning process. There are also ways to reduce the amount of motor noise a person is experiencing by adding a basic constraint, like load.

One of the benefits of adding an external force, such as load, to a movement like a squat is it decreases the number of ways a task can be done. The simple act of handing someone a weighted object and asking them to squat decreases motor noise and improves their sense of stability. The object functions as an external focal point, in addition to being extra sensory feedback. If you change the object so it's a different shape, the client will change their squatting strategy to accommodate the size of the object. How someone squats with a sandbag will look different than how the same person squats with a barbell, which will look different than squatting with a medicine ball.

Changing the shape of the load is an example of using an external constraint (weighted object) to reduce the amount of noise that occurs in a body-weight squat while still allowing a slight variation in the movement pattern because of the differing shapes. (This also makes squatting more interesting because it is a novel approach to an often-practiced task, resulting in a sense of accomplishment, so it's win-win on a number of levels.)

In individuals for whom there is anxiety around movement, picking up different-sized objects and squatting with them focuses attention. The nature of the movement makes it probable there will be the sensation of muscular work, which will cause an increase in interoception and kinesthetic awareness. The change in shapes also tends to cause a decrease in speed while the person figures out how to squat with the new weight as they move in a curious, interested way. Once the task is successfully completed, the person will likely feel a sense of empowerment and self-efficacy.

Self-Efficacy

In Chapter 2 we saw that self-efficacy is an individual's beliefs that an action will lead to a desired result. When someone has low self-efficacy, they may feel higher amounts of anxiety. They may also avoid situations they perceive as threatening (Morales-Rodriguez & Perez-Marmol, 2019).

But what happens if the situation they would like to avoid is unavoidable? For instance, if someone doesn't feel competent speaking in front of a group of people, they may avoid situations that require public speaking, but if they are asked to give the maid of honor speech at their sister's wedding, the physiological response to the heightened stress might be overwhelming. This reinforces the belief ("I can't speak in front of others because I get sweaty palms and can't formulate two sentences") and leads to more avoidance.

One of the proposed sources of self-efficacy is mastery of experience. When you attempt challenging tasks and succeed most of the time, you begin to believe your behavior does, indeed, lead to the outcome you desire. Individuals with high levels of self-efficacy view failure as a temporary setback. Instead of avoiding situations that involve public speaking, for instance, someone with high self-efficacy would take an online course or practice with a small group of friends. Persevering and working towards their goals demonstrates two traits that are hugely beneficial for mental health: adaptability and resiliency (Malik, 2013).

Resistance training positively impacts self-efficacy in a number of ways. Research has found that older adults who participate in resistance training programs experience improvements in self-efficacy, overall well-being, and view of self (Dionigi, 2007). Mastery of the physical self, for example learning how to lift progressively heavier objects or develop control over how the body responds to gravity in a variety of positions, carries over into other aspects of life. It becomes easier to fail if you know you will eventually succeed; this is important to remember throughout the lifespan. If an 82-year-old discovers they are still able to improve their physical strength, they are reminded that they are still capable of learning.

Neuroplasticity and Skeletal Plasticity

Implementing a resistance training program is largely dependent on an individual's goals (what they want to do) and what they are currently doing. We will look more at specific strength interventions in Chapter 7 when we explore practical application of concepts, but it's important to have a basic idea of how skeletal muscle works.

Skeletal muscle is malleable—capable of remodeling its structure based on the demands imposed upon it (Fluck, 2006). Variables that affect how skeletal muscle remodels include muscular force, endurance, and contractile velocity. In a strength setting, this translates into how much external load is being used and how many times the contraction occurs. External load is a fancy way of saying the amount of weight lifted. The number of contractions performed is often referred to as repetitions, or reps for short.

Activities that require lots of contractions over a sustained period of time, like walking or distance running, cause cellular changes that enable efficient oxygen delivery and metabolic efficiency. The contractile character of the muscle fibers may shift towards a slow type of muscle fiber through an exchange of components of the sarcomere, a structural unit of the muscle fiber. This is a demonstration of the SAID principle: specific adaptations to imposed demands. Regularly walking for miles doesn't require a lot of force to overcome outside resistance or the muscles to contract at a high velocity, so the muscles won't get bigger; instead, they will get better at using oxygen and contracting a lot—many times over the course of an hour.

Activities that involve high amounts of load and/or high velocity of contraction cause muscle fibers to grow and the amount of contractile proteins to increase (Hoppeler *et al.*, 2011). Another name for skeletal muscle growth is hypertrophy, and it's demonstrative of the plasticity of skeletal muscle.

Alterations in skeletal muscle structure take time, so the improvements initially seen after beginning a resistance training program aren't from a change in muscle structure but from a change in nervous system efficiency. More muscle fibers are recruited by the efferent (motor) nervous system to lift the heavy loads and motor units become synchronized, which improves coordination (Silvka *et al.*, 2008). These neurological improvements take place quickly, leading to a sense of accomplishment, a release of dopamine, and an improved sense of strength.

Movement is predicated on a number of systems in the body working together. It affects how a person feels psychologically and physically due to the complex interplay between learning, movement, and reward. Regular resistance training can influence beliefs about ability, decrease anxiety and depression, and improve coping mechanisms. Plus, it's a stepping stone to our next chapter: enriched environments.

References

Ager A.L., Borms D., Deschepper L., Dhooge R., *et al.* (2019). Proprioception: How is it affected by shoulder pain? A systematic review. Journal of Hand Therapy, 33(4), 507-516.

Aman J.E., Elangovan N., Yeh I.-L., & Konczak J. (2015). The effectiveness of proprioceptive training for improving motor function: A systematic review. Frontiers in Human Neuroscience, 8, 1075.

Buchanan T.S., Lloyd D.G., Manal K., & Besier T.F. (2004). Neuromusculoskeletal modeling: Estimation of muscle force moments and movements from measurements of neural command. Journal of Applied Biomechanics, 20(4), 367-395.

Bulbena-Cabre A., & Bulbena A. (2018). Anxiety and joint hypermobility: An unexpected association. Current Psychiatry, 17(4), 15-21.

Cimpean A., & David D. (2019). The mechanisms of pain tolerance and pain-related anxiety in acute pain. Health Psychology Open, 6(2), 1-13.

Dahlhamer J., Lucas J., Zelaya C., Nahin R., *et al.* (2018). Prevalence of chronic pain and high-impact chronic pain among adults—United States. Morbidity and Mortality Weekly Report, 67, 1001-1006.

Davis J.R., Horslen B.C., Nishikawa K., Fukushima K., *et al.* (2011). Human proprioceptive adaptation during states of height-induced fear and anxiety. Journal of Neurophysiology, 106(6), 3082-3090.

Dictionary.com (2022). Cue. Accessed on November 30, 2022 at www.dictionary.com/browse/cue.

Dionigi R. (2007). Resistance training and older adults' beliefs about psychological benefits: The importance of self-efficacy and social interaction. Journal of Sport & Exercise Psychology, 29, 723-746.

Domingues R.B., Teixeira A.L., & Domingues S.A. (2011). Physical practice is associated with less functional disability in medical students with migraines. Neurosurgery and Neuropsychiatry Archives, 69(1), 39-43.

Duquette P. (2017). Increasing our insular world view: Interoception and psychopathology for psychotherapists. Frontiers in Neuroscience, 11, 135.

Eccles J.A., Beacher F.D.C., Gray M.A., Jones C.L., *et al.* (2012). Brain structure and joint hypermobility: Relevance to the expression of psychiatric symptoms. British Journal of Psychiatry, 200(6), 508-509.

Farris C.G., Thomas J.G., Abrantes A.M., Lipton R.B., *et al.* (2019). Anxiety sensitivity and intentional avoidance of physical activity in women with probable migraine. Cephalagia: An International Journal of Headache, 39(11), 1465-1469.

Fluck M. (2006). Functional, structural and molecular plasticity of mammalian skeletal muscle in response to exercise stimuli. Journal of Experimental Biology, 209, 2239-2248.

Franchi M.V., Reeves N.D., & Narici M.V. (2017). Skeletal muscle remodeling in response to eccentric vs. concentric loading: Morphological, molecular, and metabolic adaptations. Frontiers in Physiology, 8, 447.

Gordon B.R., McDowell C.P., Lyons M., & Herring M.P. (2017). The effects of resistance exercise training on anxiety: A meta-analysis and meta-regression analysis of randomized controlled trials. Sports Medicine, 47(12), 2521-2532.

Guillamo E., Barbany J.R., Blazquez A., Delicado M.C., Ventura J.L., & Javierre C. (2016). Physical effects of a reconditioning programme in a group of chronic fatigue syndrome patients. Journal of Sports Medicine and Physical Fitness, 56(5), 579-586.

Hoppeler H., Baum O., Lurman G., & Mueller M. (2011). Molecular mechanisms of muscle plasticity with exercise. Comprehensive Physiology, 1(3), 1383-1412.

Iannello P., Mottini A., Tirelli S., Riva S., & Antonietti A. (2017). Ambiguity and uncertainty tolerance, need for cognition, and their association with stress. A study among Italian practicing physicians. Medical Education Online, 22(1), 1-10.

Ille A., Selin I., Do M-C., & Thon B. (2013). Attentional focus effects on spring start performance as a function of skill level. Journal of Sports Science, 31(15), 1705-1712.

Kawashima S., Ueki Y., Kato T., Matsukawa N., *et al.* (2012). Changes in striatal dopamine release associated with human motor-skill acquisition. PLOS ONE, 7(2), 1-9, e31728.

Kumar B., & Lenert P. (2017). Joint hypermobility syndrome: Recognizing a commonly overlooked cause of chronic pain. American Journal of Medicine, 130(6), 640-647.

Malik A. (2013). Efficacy, hope, optimism and resilience at workplace: Positive organizational behavior. International Journal of Scientific and Research Publications, 3(10), 1-4.

Manohar S.G., Chong T.T.-J., Apps M.A.J., Batia A., *et al.* (2015). Reward pays the cost of noise reduction in motor and cognitive control. Current Biology, 25(13), 1707-1716.

Marri K., & Swaminathan R. (2016). Analysis of concentric and eccentric contractions in biceps brachii muscles using surface electromyography signals and multi fractal analysis. Proceedings of the Institution of Mechanical Engineers Part H, Journal of Engineering in Medicine, 230(9), 829-839.

Mehling W.E., Acree M., Stewart A., Silas J., & Jones A. (2018). The Multidimensional Assessment of Interceptive Awareness, Version 2 (MAIA-2). PLOS ONE, 13(12), 1-20.

Mills S.E.E., Nicolson K.P., & Smith B.H. (2019). Chronic pain: A review of its epidemiology and associated factors in population-based studies. British Journal of Anesthesia, 123(2), 273-283.

Morales-Rodriguez F.M., & Perez-Marmol J.M. (2019). The role of anxiety, coping strategies, and emotional intelligence on general perceived self-efficacy in university students. Frontiers in Psychology, 10, 1689.

Olguin H.J., Guzman D.C., Garcia E.H., & Mejia G.B. (2015). The role of dopamine and its dysfunction as a consequence of oxidative stress. Oxidative Medicine and Cellular Longevity, 2016, 9730467.

Olugbade T., Bianchi-Berthouze N., & Williams A.C.C. (2019). The relationship between guarding, pain, and emotion. Pain Reports, 4(4), 1-6.

Ombregt L. (2013). Chapter 1, Section 5: Principles of Treatment, 83-115. In: A System of Orthopaedic Medicine. 3rd edition. London: Churchill Livingstone.

Paulus M.P. (2013). The breathing conundrum: Interoceptive sensitivity and anxiety. Depression and Anxiety, 30(4), 315-320.

Peres M.F.P., Mercante J.P.P., Lobo P.R., Kamei H., & Bigal M.E. (2017). Anxiety and depression symptoms and migraine: A symptom-based approach research. Journal of Headache and Pain, 18(1), 37.

Pollatos O., Traut-Mattausch E., Schroeder H., & Schandry R. (2007). Interoceptive awareness mediates the relationship between anxiety and the intensity of unpleasant feelings. Journal of Anxiety Disorders, 21(7), 931-943.

Rio E., van Ark M., Docking S., Moseley G.L., et al. (2017). Isometric contractions are more analgesic than isotonic contractions for patellar tendon pain: An in-season randomized clinical trial. Clinical Journal of Sports Medicine, 27(3), 253-259.

Salles J.I., Vasques B., Cossich V., Nicoliche E., et al. (2015). Strength training and shoulder proprioception. Journal of Athletic Training, 50(3), 277-280.

Scheibner H.J., Bogler C., Gleich T., Haynes J.D., & Bermpohl F. (2017). Internal and external attention and the default mode network. Neuroimage, 148, 381-389.

Seth A.K., Suzuki K., & Critcheley H.D. (2011). An interoceptive predictive coding model of conscious presence. Frontiers in Psychology, 2, 395.

Shalev I. (2018). Using motivated cue integration theory to understand a moment-by-moment transformative change: A new look at focusing technique. Frontiers in Human Neuroscience, 12, 307.

Silvka D., Raue U., Hilton C., Minchey K., & Trappe S. (2008). Single muscle fiber adaptations to resistance training in old (>80 yr) men: Evidence for limited skeletal muscle plasticity. American Journal of Physiology Regulatory, Integrative and Comparative Physiology, 295(1), R273-R280.

Staab J.P., Balaban C.D., & Furman J.M. (2013). Threat assessment and locomotion: Clinical application of an integrated model of anxiety and postural control. Seminars in Neurology, 33(3), 297-306.

Tao Y., Liu B., Zhang X., Li J., Qin W., Yu C., & Jiang T. (2015). The structural connectivity pattern of the default mode network and its association with memory and anxiety. Frontiers in Neuroanatomy, 9, 152.

Vadivelu N., Kai A.M., Kodumudi G., Babayan K., Fontes M., & Burg M.M. (2017). Pain and psychology: A reciprocal relationship. Ochsner Journal, 17(2), 173-180.

Vassend O., Roysamb E., Nielsen C.S., & Czajkowski N.O. (2018). Fatigue symptoms in relation to neuroticism, anxiety-depression, and musculoskeletal pain. A longitudinal twin study. PLOS ONE, 13(6), 1-21.

CHAPTER 4

Enriched Environments

Our ability to perceive the world around us is predicated on a variety of systems that take in information from both our external and internal environments. The basic mechanisms of these various systems and how they influence perception are stimulated by the environment around us. Before we explore the science of movement, enriched environments (EEs), and anxiety, let's discuss the senses that influence perception.

Exteroception

Exteroception provides us with information about the outside world (Fulkerson, 2014). It's also known as the body schema, and refers to the inferred knowledge of the body and how it relates to space and movement (Valenzuela-Moguillansky *et al.*, 2017). This ability exists because of the integration of the exteroceptive signals of vision, sound, and touch, and the internal signals from the vestibular system, proprioceptive systems, and voluntary motor system.

The vestibular system provides you with a sense of maintaining balance and allows rapid responses to perturbations from external or internal forces (Purves *et al.*, 2001). Have you ever caught your foot on seemingly nothing and felt yourself stumble, only to quickly recover so you could keep walking? That is your vestibular system at work. The inner ear acts like a miniature motion detector, letting the brainstem know how fast and at what angle the head and body are moving. Because it is a key component to both postural reflexes and eye movements, when your vestibular system is altered in some way, your eye movements and postural reflexes will be impacted, decreasing the accuracy of your knowledge of where your head and body are positioned in space.

Proprioception is the unconscious awareness of the body's position in space. It is an unconscious process that is informed by a number of other systems, including interoception and exteroceptive senses (Tsakiris *et al.*, 2011; Purves & Gandevia, 2012). Our ability to navigate the world without bumping into things that are out of our field of vision is the result of our proprioception.

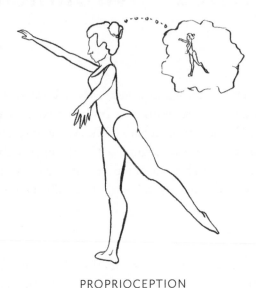

PROPRIOCEPTION

Interoception

A quick recap on interoception: it's the perception of the internal state of the body. It refers to things like visceral sensitivity, heart rate, breathing rate, and muscular tension. It influences proprioception and is influenced by signals that are interpreted as nociception.

There are two neural pathways that inform interoception. The first relays information from the skin, muscles, and joints and ends in the somatosensory cortex. It provides proprioceptive and tactile afferent information.

The second pathway relays primary visceral information to the thalamus. It provides afferent information about a variety of sensations, including pain, temperature, affective touch, and visceral sensation. What's interesting, then, is that interoceptive awareness, or the ability to detect changes in the internal state of the body, is based on a number of different sensory systems, demonstrating neatly that there is a synergistic relationship between our interpretation of our internal and external world and the input we are receiving (Ferentzi *et al.*, 2018).

Sometimes, people interpret interoceptive signals as potentially threatening or cause for concern, just like sometimes people interpret muscular sensations as potentially harmful. This is called interoceptive sensitivity and differs from interoceptive awareness, which is characterized as the ability to interpret accurately the body's physiological condition. While interceptive awareness is associated with attention regulation and acceptance and can be used to disengage from negative thoughts by interrupting the default mode network, interoceptive sensitivity is associated with hypervigilance and catastrophizing. In fact, heightened sensitivity to the physiological state of the ANS may accompany increased ANS reactivity and a decrease in pain tolerance (Hanley *et al.*, 2017; Pollatos *et al.*, 2012).

Nociception

"Nociception" is a term that refers to the neural process of encoding and processing harmful stimuli. Pain is an aspect of somatic sensation and is defined as a complex interplay of unpleasant sensory, emotional, and cognitive experiences stimulated by the perception of tissue damage. The perception of tissue damage may be due to actual tissue damage or it may be due to a perceived threat to the tissue. Pain is manifested by specific autonomic, psychological, and behavioral reactions (Dubin & Patapoutian, 2010). Pain is complex, multi-factorial, and an aspect of interoception; to recap: nociception is a specific response to potentially harmful stimuli.

Nociceptors are specialized sensory neurons that let us know when there are dangerous changes in temperature, pressure, and injury-related chemicals. It takes a lot to trigger a nociceptive response, unlike the neurons related to other senses such as vision, smell, and taste, which are highly sensitive to stimulus. Another way to say this is the afferent neurons associated with vision, smell, and taste are low threshold, while nociceptors are high-threshold neurons. Interestingly, nociceptor activity doesn't necessarily lead to the perception of pain. Pain is multi-factorial and many different factors interact to cause the sensation of pain; as a result, it is considered highly subjective and individual.

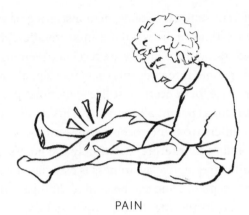

PAIN

Like all neurons, nociceptors are plastic. This means they don't return to their normal, high-threshold function after damage has occurred. They become more sensitive, and researchers report that after injury there is often a reduction in the amount of stimulus required for them to fire. This is called sensitization, and usually happens during the inflammatory phase of healing (Reichling & Levine, 2009). From a healing perspective, this increased sensitivity is good—it reminds the organism (the person healing) to protect the area, promoting a successful outcome.

Things go awry when the receptors remain sensitive after healing has occurred. This can lead to non-threatening stimuli causing pain, a condition referred to as allodynia (Sneddon, 2017). It can also result in stimuli that were slightly painful before the injury becoming extremely painful after the initial injury has healed. This is called hyperalgesia.

Imagine that you have a shoulder injury from a fall. The fall was months ago, your doctor says your shoulder is fine, but every time you try and put weight on your hand, your shoulder loudly protests. That is allodynia.

Now imagine that before the fall, you would get a small pinching sensation in the front of your shoulder when you reached your arm up overhead, towards the midline of the body. It didn't bother you, but it was something that you noticed. Since the fall, that same movement causes a sharp, intense sensation. The doctor continues to tell you everything is healed and there is nothing structurally wrong with your shoulder, yet the intensity of sensation when you attempt to lift your arm overhead towards the middle of your body suggests otherwise. This is hyperalgesia.

The brain has the ability to dial sensation from nociception up or down depending on what is happening. When sensation from nociception is dialed down because survival or homeostasis needs to be maintained, this means an analgesic effect has occurred.

Let's say you are trail running in the middle of the night and you cut your shin on a shrub with thorns. Chances are you won't notice the cut until after you are finished running. Why?

Running is a stressor that causes an uptick in SNS activity. The act of running signals that there might be something to run from. Your nervous system ensures that you make it away from the fire or to the crying baby by producing endogenous opioids that act as natural pain-killers throughout the nervous system. Voila! Pain from the cut doesn't register, and unless you notice the blood running down your leg, you will be pain free until you come to a stop.

It's possible you have witnessed this at some point in your life, for example when a child who is playing with friends cuts himself and doesn't notice until he sees the blood after he is done playing, or an animal fighting with another animal experiences a blow to the leg that doesn't appear to faze it until after the fight is over and its limb suddenly appears to give out. We are hardwired for survival; survival doesn't always have time for us to experience, feel, and nurture our injuries.

Conversely, chronic stress can increase the perception of pain. Researchers suggest that when cortisol secretion is intensified as a result of psychological and emotional stress, the result is a sensitized stress response that kicks in a little too readily. Prolonged stress may result in cortisol dysfunction, widespread inflammation, and pain (Hannibal & Bishop, 2014). (For a refresher on how cortisol works, please refer to Chapter 1.)

Chronic stress happens for a myriad of reasons. Some factors include rumination and anxiety, lack of social support (Ozbay et al., 2007), and insomnia (Han et al., 2012). While it's difficult to know if chronic stress causes the lack of social support and/or sleep deprivation, or if the lack of social support and/or lack of sleep cause chronic stress, it is important to note that chronic stress affects several aspects of an individual's life.

And so can the perception of pain. Unfortunately, it's not as cut and dry as "If it hurts, avoid it at all possible costs," or "No pain, no gain." Have you ever taken a step, had a twinge in your knee, and then taken another step, only to have the pain disappear? When there is heightened sensitivity in the nervous system, sometimes little twinges happen. This doesn't indicate tissue damage or movement that should be avoided. Often, in a movement setting, if someone feels sensation that is perceived as muscular pain during a movement skill, if the individual is instructed to alter the movement slightly, the pain will disappear. Whether that's because the shift in loading is enough to decrease nociceptor sensitivity, or slightly shifting the perspective of the movement downregulates the nervous system in some way, I'm not sure, but the point is, if pain is described as muscular, vague, or like a wandering gnome, it's worthwhile to approach movement curiously and see if there are positions and movements that are pain free. This helps empower the client, making them feel more confident in their physical abilities.

If, on the other hand, the pain is described as burning, sharp, tingling, or inside the joint, movements that exacerbate the pain should be avoided. This is where it can be helpful to direct attention outside the self, finding externally based actions that don't exacerbate feelings of discomfort and that allow the individual to self-organize. One way to do this is through EEs.

Enriched Environments

EEs are characterized in animal studies as environments where animals have space, access to sensory-stimulating objects, and opportunities for physical activity and social interaction (Ball et al., 2019). Animals that live in EEs show a reduction in emotional reactivity and abnormal behavior, and experience improved cognitive functioning. One of the main goals of EEs is to stimulate curiosity; curiosity enhances learning and memory.

What constitutes an EE for humans is up for debate. Research on the topic is in its infancy, though a 2017 study found that living near forests may create more balance in the amygdala, the small, almond-shaped portion of the temporal lobe in the brain that modulates emotion-regulated behavior (Kuhn et al., 2017). The amygdala is most often implicated in fear response; in a review of 55 imaging studies examining the functional neuroanatomy of emotion, 25 found amygdala activation to fear-based stimuli and four found activation to positive stimuli (Ressler, 2010). When part of the amygdala is removed, patients demonstrate deficits in fear-conditioned startle responses, suggesting that the amygdala plays an important role in fear response regulation (ibid.; Kuhn et al., 2017).

When there is an unexpected stimulus, such as a loud noise, the pupils dilate and muscles contract (Nijhuis *et al.*, 2007). Your eyes orient your head to the direction of the noise in order to determine whether the sound is an actual threat. Though desensitization to that specific sound as a form of potential stress can occur, you will still blink and experience increased arousal when an auditory stimulus is present (de Haan *et al.*, 2018). An auditory stimulus is something like a siren, a door slamming shut, or the unexpected rev of a motorcycle. Cities, while enriching on a social level, have large amounts of unanticipated noise, which may translate into increased amounts of arousal. This isn't necessarily bad, but when you are assessing how to create an EE for a client, using noise that doesn't increase arousal may benefit learning.

Remember, noise is an auditory sense, so it can be used as a way to add to the environment. Music, specifically, is believed to be a feature of the world that is universal, a form of creativity that was meant to be shared with others. The response to the music is movement that occurs through dancing to the beat of time (Trimble & Hesdorffer, 2017). In fact, it has been suggested that music gave us a way to express feelings and emotions before words.

Dance is a physical expression that occurs as a result of the feelings evoked by music. Movement, though it appears continuous, is actually based on the perception of tasks and events (Blasing, 2015). The sensory input you receive and information you have learned previously naturally segments movement into parts, allowing the neuromuscular system to anticipate and react to upcoming information. If I asked you to play a song you know well and move around until the song ends, you would phrase movements that are familiar to match the phrasing of the music, linking it together in a way that appears continuous.

If the movement in response to music is done with others, this adds to the environment. Suddenly, there is a social component and attention shifts to the connection with the other person. There are different ways movement can be performed with another person, including choreographed sequencing where everyone performs the same steps, but for the purposes of discussing creating EEs, let's focus on movements where one person leads and one person follows.

In many forms of dance or partner movement, the leader role is fluid, depending on the context. Research performed on experienced tango dancers found that leading movement activated the areas of the brain associated with motor planning, navigation, sequencing, action monitoring, and error correction, making it an internally driven process. Following was a more externally driven process, activating the areas of the brain associated with somatosensation, proprioception, motion tracking, social cognition, and outcome monitoring (Chauvigne *et al.*, 2018).

Collective dance improvisation (CDI) is a form of dance that involves at least two people performing movements that are based on (and regulated by) the experiences that arise from moving together. The experience can be framed as a game, or game play, which is defined by philosopher Bernard Suits (Suits *et al.*, 2014) as "the voluntary attempt to overcome unnecessary obstacles." Games can have an end goal, such as in a sporting event, or they can be performed as a way to explore a process. Games have conditions or constraints that limit which options are used; in the context of CDI, solutions are determined based on the movement of your partner (or partners, if there are more than two people dancing together). Navigating the obstacles that arise while negotiating movement with another person leads to a kinesthetic experience of movement, specifically through internal senses (muscles, joints, viscera, and vestibular system) and external senses (visual and auditory systems). The environment, then, becomes enriching on a number of levels, utilizing a variety of senses to create realistic solutions to the questions posed by the game (Himberg *et al.*, 2018).

The concepts of music, game play, and partner interaction can be used in a variety of ways in a movement setting. The practical applications of these concepts will be discussed in Chapter 9, but take a moment to consider open-ended movement games where there is no winner or loser. What do they look like? When was the last time you participated in one? Were you always able to complete the task successfully, or was there an element of challenge? Did it feel like "exercise"?

Dance movement psychotherapy (DMT) is a form of therapy influenced by modern dance and somatic lineages developed over the last century (Payne, 2017). Elements of DMT can be used to develop interoceptive sensing and body awareness, specifically proprioception, empathy, and attunement. A 2019 meta-analysis on DMT and dance interventions found that improvements in quality of life, decreases in depression and anxiety, and improvement in motor skills (Koch *et al.*, 2019). (Dance interventions are believed to share therapeutic mechanisms with DMT and are defined as various dance styles, such as ballroom dancing and folk dance.) Creative arts therapies have established five different mechanisms that describe why they are effective: pleasure/play and a non-goal orientation, experiencing body-mind unity, emotion expression/regulation and social interaction, experiencing agency/self-efficacy and activity, and creation (*ibid.*).

Providing environments where individuals use both their minds and their bodies to problem solve enhances the client's experience. It enables clients to experience the act of moving in a way that becomes about something bigger than burning calories or looking a specific way. This form of movement creates a sense of wholeness and, for even the briefest moment, brings the client into the present, away from feelings of anxiousness or worry and gives them an opportunity to explore a deeper connection of embodiment.

The Physiological Benefits of Enriched Environments

There are a number of neurological changes associated with EEs, including morphological, molecular, and physiological changes to the motor and sensory cortices in the brains of young and adult animals. Cortical thickness increases and dendritic branches increase, and there are more synapses per neuron in animals raised in EEs compared with animals raised in standard conditions (Engineer *et al.*, 2004).

The experience-dependent plasticity that occurs during repeated exposure to an EE has positive effects on a variety of brain disorders, including Huntington's disease, Parkinson's, Alzheimer's, amyotrophic lateral sclerosis (ALS), and Down's syndrome (Nithianantharajah & Hannan, 2006). What constitutes an EE is debatable, though it's worth noting that living in strictly urban environments is associated with lower grey-matter volume and higher amygdala activity, indicating that city living may increase an individual's risk of chronic stress. Living near a forest may actually improve the integrity of the amygdala, enabling people to appropriately respond to stress and adequately recover once the stress has dissipated (Kuhn *et al.*, 2017). Urban environments may be linked to chronic stress not only because of the large amounts of stimulation, but also the lack of interpersonal space. This is consistent with what researchers have found in animal studies. Having space is good for the brain (and gives you more opportunities to move).

It has been suggested that the mammalian brain evolved as the natural environment developed (Lambert *et al.*, 2016). Rats exposed to naturally enriched environments filled with natural stimuli and rats exposed to an artificially enriched environment with man-made stimuli both exhibit less anxiety to a novel stimulus than rats placed in a standard environment with only food and water; the naturally enriched rats, however, exhibit less behavior associated with anxiety when exposed to the smell of a predator than rats in the artificially enriched environment or the standard environment (*ibid.*).

What's interesting about this is the naturally enriched environment rats are exhibiting higher thresholds to stressful events, which suggests an increase in resilience. When you think about how this translates to people, people who are prone to anxiety are going to find anything new stressful (this includes exercise/movement programs). People who have a higher anxiety tolerance may find new experiences and stimuli interesting or a challenge. This is one of the reasons two people can be exposed to the same stimuli and have very different experiences.

Confession: I find traditional gym settings both uninviting and overly stimulating (I usually carve out a small space in the corner, away from the machines, with my headphones on and the free weights I want). It's entirely possible I am either overly sensitive or an anomaly (or both), but if gyms are the adult equivalent of an EE, offering alternatives for more sensitive people may make exercise more inviting. Designing movement spaces that have open space, objects that spark interest and can be used to provide context to movement, and more natural light may make exercise more appealing for this subset of the population. An alternative for those who don't have access to indoor space because of cost is to use natural green spaces and parks for outdoor classes which, as you just learned, may be a great way to introduce movement in a more natural environment. And if you don't have access to outdoor settings, adding plants and/or natural landscapes to your working space can provide visual input reminiscent of nature.

This isn't to say the traditional gym environment doesn't work. It works for a lot of people really well—in fact, many people thrive off the energy. But if you are working with individuals who are more sensitive to their environment, it's important to remember that changing it may create an experience that is more conducive for consistency and learning.

A quick recap on the effects of prolonged stress on the brain: chronic stress causes changes in the structure and function of the hippocampus, including reduced long-term potentiation, less generation of nerve cells in the brain, less ability to navigate the environment and retain information about the environment, and impairments in working memory. EEs positively impact the structure and function of the hippocampus through improved memory and increased nerve-cell generation in the hippocampus. In fact, when chronically stressed rats were placed in an EE for six hours a day over the course of ten days, the effect of chronic stress on anxiety behavior was significantly reduced, completely restoring cognitive function (Bhagya *et al.*, 2017).

A similar reversal was seen when infant rats that were separated from their mothers for three hours a day over the course of 12 days were exposed to music. The rats originally demonstrated a decrease in sociability and an increase in behaviors associated with depression and anxiety; musical enrichment reversed these effects (Papadakakis *et al.*, 2019). (For those of you wondering, the rats were exposed to Mozart. It would be interesting to see if the results were the same if the rats were exposed to, say, Metallica or Jay-Z.) I am not suggesting that you play Mozart while you are working with your clients; however, it is important to remember that everything is a source of stimulation. How something is perceived and whether it can be considered enriching depends on a variety of factors, including the emotional state of the client.

The Vestibular System and Its Role in Enriched Environments

The vestibular system works with the proprioceptive system and the visual system to maintain balance. It has been shown to affect anxiety and stress levels in several ways (Saman *et al.*, 2012). How they are correlated is unclear, though there may be a connection between the stress hormones cortisol and corticosterone and their ability to bind to another neuron. Stress hormones may also affect inner ear function by impacting ionic homeostasis in the inner ear.

What all of this means is stress may impact your balance. Is the inverse of this also true? Does balance affect stress?

It turns out that it may. Research suggests a link between poor balance and symptoms related to anxiety; when children with balance dysfunctions were compared with a control group (children with no balance problems), they rated higher in anxiety and lower in self-esteem (Bart *et al.*, 2009). Fortunately, when children with balance dysfunction were placed in a 12-week balance intervention, their balance improved, and so did their self-esteem, while their anxiety decreased (*ibid.*). In the elderly, anxiety and dizziness are common complaints, making it difficult to know if anxiety is causing dizziness or dizziness is causing anxiety. Interestingly, anxiety and dizziness share some neural pathways. In fact, one hypothesis regarding the connection between them is that signals from the inner ear are misinterpreted by the CNS, causing the CNS to send out a warning signal of an imminent threat; this, in turn, heightens anxiety (Carmeli, 2015).

Fortunately, EEs stimulate the vestibular system in a number of ways, and because of the brain's plasticity and ability to remodel at any age, balance can improve. In animal models, active training and physical activity induce structural and functional reorganization of neurons; they also improve behavior and cognition (Lacour & Bernard-Demanze, 2015). Active training means the animal is engaged in what it is doing; in humans, this is akin to being focused on the task and mentally engaged, which is exactly what EEs do—provide an opportunity to focus and engage.

Integrating movement environments for the vestibular system requires utilizing the eyes (Anastasopoulos *et al.*, 2019). The vestibule-ocular reflex (VOR) allows the recovery of gaze and visual input when the head changes position. This allows the gaze to feel stable even if it is shifting. Therefore, using gaze (and a change in head position) during movement will train the VOR. This can be done in a variety of ways, but since this particular section is on EEs, we will focus on how using the environment can stimulate (and train) the VOR.

When there are obstacles to navigate, the change in body position to get around (or through, or over) the obstacles requires input from the systems that comprise balance. When there are objects to reach for or catch, the balance system is again stimulated. Finally, if there is an element of game play as defined above, either with another person or through use of a constraint, the balance system is stimulated. Inviting clients to participate in situations that don't have clear solutions, where attention needs to be focused and multiple senses must be used, challenges the client to be present and emphasizes balance and a sense of stability. This will, at least for a moment, reduce anxious thoughts and interrupt the default mode network.

Proprioception and Enriched Environments

Proprioception happens unconsciously and is influenced by interoception; in fact, some researchers view sensations from the musculoskeletal system as interoceptive senses. This makes sense when you think of pain as being an aspect of interoception. The perception of pain is, as discussed above, based on an individual's interpretation of sensation. Often, when I ask people to describe the sensation of pain, they describe a vague muscular sensation of tightness or a dull ache. This implies they are receiving afferent input from the musculoskeletal system that is being interpreted as harmful.

The term "proprioception" was first introduced by Sir Charles Scott Sherrington, a neuroscientist in the early 1900s who made several contributions to our understanding of the nervous system and how the mind and the body are connected physiologically. He coined the term in 1893 and went on to make several other original contributions to the understanding of neurons, including the description of synaptic transmission (Pearce, 2004).

If your environment is predictable, your proprioception will be less developed than if you have a more sensory-rich environment. It has been argued that the muscle spindles are the main source of proprioceptive information, with cutaneous receptors playing a supporting role in proprioception (Proske, 2015). Muscle spindles are located within the body of the muscle and detect changes in muscle length. Cutaneous receptors are located in the skin.

Mechanoreceptors embedded in joint capsules also play a role in proprioception, providing the CNS with information about joint position and joint motion based on two different types of mechanoreceptors: type 1 and type 2 (Witherspoon et al., 2014).

Type 1 mechanoreceptors, or Ruffini corpuscles, are slow adapting. They respond to stimuli that are prolonged and constant, such as stretch, rotation, and compression. Type 2, or Pacinian or Krause corpuscles, are rapid adapting. They respond to the beginning and end of the stimulus.

Let's say you are sitting with your arm in an awkward position for a few minutes. The sensations that begin to arise from your arm are probably the result of the type 1 mechanoreceptors registering your position and providing afferent feedback to your CNS that says, "Hey. This is a little bit uncomfortable. Maybe you should shift."

If, on the other hand, you are rapidly swinging your arms, the CNS will register arm swinging and the change in shoulder position because of afferent feedback from type 2 mechanoreceptors. If you were asked to describe your arms at the end of the exercise, your description would likely be more robust than normal because of the recent stimulation—movement creates input. This results in more sensory information than normal, giving you a more clear image of your arm and its position in space.

Let's say you were asked to crawl over a variety of surfaces and vault over objects of different sizes and shapes. You would receive proprioceptive input from your skin as it detects the change in densities and textures, your muscles as their length/tension relationships change to move the body forward, and the joints as they change position. Additionally, because the landscape of the environment is interesting, you will utilize your eyes to help you navigate (unless you are doing this in the dark, which would heighten your proprioception to make up for the loss of vision to keep you balanced).

Proprioception can be impacted by a number of factors, including stroke, neuropathy, and age. But, due to the brain's plasticity and the ability to learn across the lifespan, EEs can lead to a dramatic improvement in proprioception (at least in animal studies).

Remember that there appears to be a correlation between balance and anxiety? The three systems that directly impact balance are the visual system, vestibular system, and proprioceptive system. These systems help you remain balanced, upright, and able to respond to perturbations (unexpected external forces). Ergo, improving proprioception will improve balance, which may lead to a reduction in anxiety. A fun and interesting way to do this is through environments that stimulate curiosity and have multiple solutions to the same task.

While the research on humans and EEs is woefully scant, I am hoping this book inspires someone to study the effects of human obstacle courses/parkour/MovNat/other modalities that utilize the environment on anxiety. In the meantime, animal studies are demonstrating promising results.

In a study (Buchhold *et al.*, 2007) of older (aged 20 months) and younger (aged three months) rats that had experienced induced stroke, the older rats showed more severe behavioral impairments and reduced functional recovery than the younger rats. When the rats were placed in an EE, the size of the infarct (the damaged area) reduced in both groups, and so did the number of proliferating astrocytes and the volume of the glial scar (both indicators of brain injury). Additionally, the EE led to significant improvements in rate and extent of recovery in the older rats.

Another study (Young *et al.*, 2015) looked at animals that were given a traumatic brain injury in the sensorimotor cortex and then placed in EEs. These animals were compared with animals that had experienced the same injury and been given nerve growth factor through the nose. (Nerve growth factor is a protein that naturally occurs in the brain and has been found to improve motor and cognitive function after traumatic brain injuries.) EEs were found to be effective for motor function recovery, while nerve growth factor was not, suggesting that placing animals in an EE is a more effective way to improve motor function than giving them nerve growth factor.

Finally, a third study (Hakon *et al.*, 2017) examined mice that, again, were subjected to stroke and then placed either in a standard housing environment or an EE. It turns out that spontaneous recovery of sensorimotor function post-stroke is associated with changes that can actually be seen in the brain in resting-state functional connectivity. The EE included multisensory stimulation, which means different textures were included. EE cages contained things like tubes, chains, ladders, toys, and platforms that were at varying levels. The EE mice had partial restoration of their resting-state functional connectivity between the hemispheres of their brains in several motor regions that weren't affected during stroke.

What all of these studies suggest is that exposure to appropriately stimulating environments leads to changes that are bigger than simply improved proprioception and balance (though that is certainly import-ant). They elicit changes in the brain. Granted, this was after traumatic brain injuries or events, but it would stand to reason that in healthy brains, exposure to EEs would improve proprioception and cognitive function on some level.

The Coach's Role as Part of the Enriched Environment

It's important to note that the person guiding the session is an aspect of an EE. How you instruct and how you relate to the person with whom you are working is a social interaction. Your interaction can enrich the person's environment if you are kind and thoughtful, and choose words that make the client feel empowered and confident.

If you view your role as giving instructions without reciprocal communication from the client, you are setting up a dynamic that has a power differential. More simply, you are viewed as the expert who knows all, and the client is placed in a more submissive role, where they are expected to perform the action as instructed. This limits the client's self-efficacy and self-agency, and doesn't give them an opportunity to practice interoception or reflection.

Remember that self-agency is an individual's sense of embodiment (Gallagher & Trigg, 2016), and self-efficacy is an individual's belief in their capabilities (Tahmassian & Moghadam, 2011). Anxiety can have a negative impact on both self-agency and self-efficacy, so if your goal is to provide an experience that is enriching and positively impacts an individual's sense of resiliency and self, it is important the relationship doesn't feel one-sided. There can be moments of reflection or invitations to allow the client to move in a more organic and less structured way to increase empowerment (examples will given in Chapter 9 when we examine practical applications of game play in a movement setting).

Another way to invite reflection is to ask clients what they are experiencing or ask them to describe how they are performing a skill. The ability to accurately gauge an internal experience requires interoceptive accuracy, which means that the client has an accurate sense of what their perception of their internal state means. This is different than interoceptive awareness or interoceptive sensitivity, though awareness and sensitivity all influence accuracy (Forkmann et al., 2019).

A client's ability to articulate how they are performing a skill requires a high degree of kinesthetic awareness and the ability to translate that experience into words. A term that is sometimes used to define an individual's ability to use the body to solve problems, express ideas and emotion, and manipulate objects is bodily-kinesthetic intelligence (Michelaki & Bournelli, 2016). The problem with the word "intelligence" is it is often interpreted to mean an innate ability that one is born with rather than a sense that can be developed. However, like all forms of intelligence, bodily-kinesthetic intelligence can be improved upon with practice, reflection, and focused attention.

We know that aerobic exercise can give people prone to anxiety a more accurate sense of their interoceptive cues. If someone doesn't have a good gauge of what these cues mean, asking the individual to focus on them more can actually increase anxiety and/or fear around movement if the cues are misinterpreted. This can be particularly true if you are working with someone who is experiencing PTSD.

PTSD is not classified as an anxiety disorder. The DSM-5 considers it a trauma- and stress-related disorder that must include exposure to a traumatic or stressful event as an aspect of its diagnosis (American Psychiatric Association, 2013). Individuals experiencing PTSD often have changes in their bodily self-awareness and interoception. Curiously, these changes may disrupt the integration between the vestibular system and the brainstem, specifically in individuals who are categorized as dissociative, which means they feel like their bodies don't actually belong to them (Harricharan *et al.*, 2017).

Interoceptive exposure is an intervention that aims to reduce anxiety sensitivity and distress through somatic sensations. It is used to treat panic disorder, PTSD, and a range of anxiety disorders. Unfortunately, the research on the utilization of somatic techniques such as interoceptive exposure is scarce, though many researchers advocate the benefits and potential for somatic techniques to improve emotional regulation and fear related to somatic sensations (Boettcher *et al.*, 2016).

If you are not trained or licensed in somatic therapies or interoceptive exposure, asking someone with heightened interoceptive sensitivity what they are experiencing may make them feel more anxious, overloading the sensory system and negating the benefits of the reflection. It is the coach's job to observe the client, see what they are responding to, and, through active listening techniques, tap into an effective way to facilitate the client's learning.

Active Listening

According to researchers Phil Hunsaker and Tony Alessandra, people do four general types of listening: non-listening, marginal listening, evaluative listening, and active listening (Jahromi *et al.*, 2016). Active listening is considered the most effective form of listening and is based on paying complete attention to what someone is saying by listening carefully, showing interest, and not interrupting. The listener listens for content, intention, and feeling of the person speaking. This is demonstrated through asking questions and body language that signifies the speaker has something important to say. Body movement, posture, facial expression, eye contact, reflection of content, and attentive silence are all indicators that someone is actively listening.

Active listening means the coach takes an interest in the client. It also gives the client space to voice concern and/or have an active role in their program. This helps the client feel validated and empowered, both of which can positively impact program adherence. This doesn't mean that if the client dislikes a particular movement, it is avoided altogether, or that the coach doesn't offer corrections or ideas; it simply means that the relationship is more of a partnership, a quest to help the person overcome physical and emotional obstacles through a program that enhances strength, balance, and flexibility in some way. We will discuss ideas for specific coaching strategies in Chapter 6, but for now, consider your role as one that makes the client's environment enriched.

Active listening can also improve a client's satisfaction with care received, which, hypothetically anyway, may also increase adherence. In a 2020 study, a phone interview was conducted with 97 patients receiving care for chronic pain. The number one factor related to satisfaction with care was the provider listening (Grub *et al.*, 2020).

Finally, one of the things an intelligently designed EE does (other than spark interest or curiosity) is provide scalable opportunities to learn. While a novel stimulus may cause dopamine to be released and flood the system, it can also cause activation of the SNS if the novel stimulus is perceived as threatening. In a movement setting, what this generally translates to is an exercise or skill that is perceived by the client as too challenging for their current level.

This, of course, gets tricky. The goal of the coach is to coax the client to try new things, and sometimes, as the outsider looking in, you know the client is capable of the task you are suggesting, but the client sees the task as an impossibility. If you have already established a relationship built on trust and you present the task in a way that reduces the client's internal sense of fear, the client will be more willing to try. When they are successful, they not only will feel a sense of accomplishment, they also will have strengthened their trust in both you and their abilities.

This doesn't mean you should discredit the client's concerns; rather, through active listening and empathic communication, you can find ways to appropriately challenge the client's preconceived notions of what they are capable of.

EXERCISE

The next time you are in the space in which you work, pick one object you use with clients regularly. Set a timer for ten minutes. Explore ways to use the object that differ from how you usually use it. I encourage you to look at the familiar as though it were brand new and you have no idea how it works. It is through embodying these ideas in your own practice that you will be able to relate better to the experience of your client and maintain a high level of engagement with your work, both of which will improve your client's experience.

References

American Psychiatric Association (2013). Diagnostic and Statistical Manual of Mental Disorders. 5th edition. https://doi.org/10.1176/appi.books.9780890425596.

Anastasopoulos D., Ziavra N., & Bronstein A.M. (2019). Large gaze shift generation while standing: The role of the vestibular system. Journal of Neurophysiology, 122, 1928-1936.

Ball N.J., Mercado III E., & Orduna I. (2019). Enriched environments as a potential treatment for developmental disorders: A critical assessment. Frontiers in Psychology, 10, 466.

Bart O., Bar-Hai Y., Weizman E., Levin M., Sadeh A., & Mintz M. (2009). Balance treatment ameliorates anxiety and increases self-esteem in children with comorbid anxiety and balance disorder. Research in Developmental Disabilities, 30(3), 486-495.

Bhagya V.R., Srikumar B.N., Veena J., & Shankaranarayana R.B.S. (2017). Short-term exposure to enriched environment rescues chronic stress-induced impaired hippocampal synaptic plasticity, anxiety, and memory deficits. Journal of Neuroscience Research, 95(8), 1602-1610.

Blasing B.E. (2015). Segmentation of dance movement: Effects of expertise, visual familiarity, motor experience, and music. Frontiers in Psychology, 5, 1500.

Boettcher H., Brake C.A., & Barlow D.H. (2016). Origins and outlook of interoceptive exposure. Journal of Behavior Therapy and Experimental Psychiatry, 53, 41-51.

Buchhold B., Mogoanta L., Suofu Y., Hamm A., et al. (2007). Environmental enrichment improves functional and neuropathological indices following stroke in young and aged rats. Restorative Neurology and Neuroscience, 25(5-6), 467-484.

Carmeli E. (2015). Anxiety in the elderly can be a vestibular problem. Frontiers in Public Health, 3, 216.

Chauvigne L.A.S., Belyk M., & Brown S. (2018). Taking two to tango: fMRI analysis of improvised joint action with physical contact. PLOS ONE, 13(1), 1-23.

de Haan M.I.C., van Well S., Visser R.M., Scholte S., van Wingen G.A., & Kindt M. (2018). The influence of acoustic startle probes on fear learning in humans. Scientific Reports, 8, 14552.

Dubin A.E., & Patapoutian A. (2010). Nociceptors: The sensors of the pain pathway. Journal of Clinical Investigation, 120(11), 3760-3772.

Engineer N.D., Percaccion C.R., Pandya P.K., Moucha R., Rathbun D.L., & Kilgard M.P. (2004). Environmental enrichment improves response strength, threshold, selectivity, and latency of auditory cortex neurons. Journal of Neurophysiology, 92, 73-82.

Ferentzi E., Bogdany T., Szabolcs Z., Csala B., Horváth A., & Köteles F. (2018). Multichannel investigation of interoception: Sensitivity is not a generalizable feature. Frontiers in Human Neuroscience, 12, 223.

Forkmann T., Volz-Sidiropoulou E., Helbing T., Druke B., et al. (2019). Sense it and use it: Interoceptive accuracy and sensibility in suicide ideators. BMC Psychiatry, 19, 334.

Fulkerson M. (2014). Rethinking the senses and their interaction: The case for sensory pluralism. Frontiers in Psychology, 5, 1426.

Gallagher S., & Trigg D. (2016). Agency and anxiety: Delusions of control and loss of control in schizophrenia and agoraphobia. Frontiers in Human Neuroscience, 10, 459.

Grub I., Firemark A., McMullen C.K., Mayhew M., & DeBar L.L. (2020). Satisfaction with primary care providers and health care services among patients with chronic pain: A mixed-methods study. Journal of General Internal Medicine, 35(10), 190-197.

Hakon J., Quattromani M.J., Sjolund C., Tomasevic G., et al. (2017). Multisensory stimulation improves functional recovery and resting-state T functional connectivity in the mouse brain after stroke. NeuroImage: Clinical, 17(2018), 717-730.

Han K.S., Kim L., & Shim I. (2012). Stress and sleep disorder. Experimental Neurobiology, 21(4), 141-150.

Hanley A.W., Mehling W.E., & Garland E.L. (2017). Holding the body in mind: Interoceptive awareness, dispositional mindfulness and psychological well-being. Journal of Psychosomatic Research, 99, 13-20.

Hannibal K.E., & Bishop M.D. (2014). Chronic stress, cortisol dysfunction, and pain: A psychoneuroendocrine rationale for stress management in pain rehabilitation. Physical Therapy, 94(12), 1816-1825.

Harricharan S., Nicholson A.A., Densmore M., Theberge J., et al. (2017). Sensory overload and imbalance: Resting state vestibular connectivity in PTSD and its dissociative subtype. Neuropsychologia, 106, 169-178.

Himberg T., Laroche J., Bige R., Buchkowski M., & Bachrach A. (2018). Coordinated interpersonal behavior in collective dance improvisation: The aesthetics of kinaesthetic togetherness. Behavioral Sciences, 8(2), 1-26.

Jahromi V.K., Tabatabaee S.S., Abdar Z.E., & Rajabi M. (2016). Active listening: The key of successful communication in hospital managers. Electronic Physician, 8(3), 2123-2128.

Koch S.C., Riege R.F.F., Tisborn K., Biondo J., Martin L., & Beelman A. (2019). Effects of dance movement therapy and dance on health-related physiological outcomes: A meta-analalysis. Frontiers in Psychology, 10, 1806.

Kuhn S., Duzel S., Elbich P., Krekel C., et al. (2017). In search of features that constitute an "enriched environment" in humans: Associations between geographical properties and brain structure. Scientific Reports, 7(1), 1-8.

Lacour M., & Bernard-Demanze L. (2015). Interaction between vestibular compensation mechanisms and vestibular rehabilitation therapy: 10 recommendations for optimal functional recovery. Frontiers in Neurology, 5, 285.

Lambert K., Hyer M., Bardi M., Rzucidlo A., et al. (2016). Natural-enriched environments lead to enhanced environmental engagement and neurobiological resilience. Neuroscience, 330, 386-394.

Michelaki E., & Bournelli P. (2016). The development of bodily-kinesthetic intelligence through creative dance for preschool students. Journal of Educational and Social Research, 6(3), 23-32.

Nijhuis L.B.O., Janssen L., Bloem B.R., van Dijk J.G., et al. (2007). Choice reaction times for human head rotations are shortened by startling acoustic stimuli, irrespective of stimulus direction. Journal of Physiology, 584(1), 97-109.

Nithianantharajah J., & Hannan A.J. (2006). Enriched environments, experience-dependent plasticity and disorders of the nervous system. Nature Reviews Neuroscience, 7, 697-709.

Ozbay F., Johnson D.C., Dimoulas E., Morgan III C.A., Charney D., & Southwick S. (2007). Social support and resilience to stress. From neurobiology to clinical practice. Psychiatry, 4(5), 35-40.

Papadakakis A., Sidropoulou K., & Panagis G. (2019). Music exposure attenuates anxiety- and depression-like behaviors and increases hippocampal spine density in male rats. Behavioural Brain Research. doi: 10.1016/j.bbr.2019.112023.

Payne H. (2017). Essentials of Dance Movement Therapy: International Perspectives on Theory, Research, and Practice. Routledge: London.

Pearce J.M.S. (2004). Sir Charles Scott Sherrington (1885-1952) and the synapse. Journal of Neurology, Neurosurgery, & Psychiatry, 75(4), 544.

Pollatos O., Fustos J., & Critchlet H.D. (2012). On the generalized embodiment of pain: How interoceptive sensitivity modulates cutaneous pain perception. Pain, 153(8), 1680-1686.

Proske U. (2015). The role of muscle proprioceptors in human limb position sense: A hypothesis. Journal of Anatomy, 227(2), 178-183.

Purves D., Augustine G.J., Fitzpatrick D., Katz L.C., et al. (2001). Chapter 14: The Vestibular System, 315-336. In: Neuroscience. 2nd edition. Sunderland, MA: Sinauer Associates.

Purves U., & Gandevia S.C. (2012). The proprioceptive senses: Their roles in signaling body shape, body position and movement, and muscle force. Physiological Reviews, 92(4), 1651-1697.

Reichling D.B., & Levine J.D. (2009). Critical role of nociceptor plasticity in chronic pain. Trends in Neuroscience, 32(12), 611-618.

Ressler K.J. (2010). Amygdala activity, fear, and anxiety: Modulation by stress. Biological Psychiatry, 67(12), 1117-1119.

Saman Y., Bamiou D.E., Gleeson M., & Dutia M.B. (2012). Interactions between stress and vestibular compensation—a review. Frontiers in Neurology, 3, 116.

Sneddon L.U. (2017). Comparative physiology of nociception and pain. Physiology, 33(1), 63-73.

Suits B., Hurka T., & Newfeld F. (2014). The Grasshopper: Games, Life, and Utopia. 3rd edition. Tonawanda, NY: Broadview Press.

Tahmassian K., & Moghadam N.J. (2011). Relationship between self-efficacy and symptoms of anxiety, depression, worry and social avoidance in a normal sample of students. Iranian Journal of Psychiatry and Behavioral Sciences, 5(2), 91-98.

Trimble M., & Hesdorffer D. (2017). Music and the brain: The neuroscience of music and musical appreciation. BJPsych International, 14(2), 28-31.

Tsakiris M., Tajadura-Jimenez A., & Costantini M. (2011). Just a heartbeat away from one's body: Interoceptive sensitivity predicts malleability of body-representations. Proceedings of the Royal Society B., 278(1717), 2470-2476.

Valenzuela-Moguillansky C., Reyes-Reyes A., & Gaete M.I. (2017). Exteroceptive and interoceptive body-self awareness in fibromyalgia patients. Frontiers in Human Neuroscience, 11, 117.

Witherspoon J.W., Smirnov I.V., & McIff T.E. (2014). Neuroanatomical distribution of mechanoreceptors in the human cadaveric shoulder capsule and labrum. Journal of Anatomy, 225(3), 337-345.

Young J., Pionk T., Hiatt I., Geeck K., & Smith J.S. (2015). Environmental enrichment aides in functional recovery following unilateral controlled cortical impact of the forelimb sensorimotor area however intranasal administration of nerve growth factor does not. Brain Research Bulletin, 115, 17-22.

CHAPTER 5

The Value of Gentle Movement

A client I hadn't seen in a while contacted me recently. She'd injured her collarbone trying to do a pull-up during the Covid lockdown. Her husband, a pain doctor, had suggested that she see me for some ideas on how to restore movement to the area without aggravating it.

We did gentle, focused movement that incorporated specific mobility throughout the spine and shoulder blades. I chose movements that provided lots of sensory feedback so she would feel more grounded and centered, and I borrowed from a variety of restorative modalities, including Feldenkrais and Tai Chi.

By the end of the session, she felt better. She texted me the next day, saying she couldn't explain it, but after two months of persistent discomfort, the pain had subsided substantially. She had slept much better and she felt hopeful that maybe her collarbone would actually heal.

So far in the book, we have discussed the benefits of exercise and EEs, and how those things impact mental health. As you learned, EEs provide context for movement, and utilize multiple senses and focused attention. But what about moving in ways that are purposefully mindful, such as in yoga, Tai Chi, or somatic-based practices? How do these types of modalities fit when you are designing and implementing a movement and exercise program for people with anxiety, depression, or trauma?

It's worth noting that any form of movement, including traditional exercise modalities, can be taught in a way that connects the mind with the body. We will discuss this more in Chapter 6, but for now, just know that if someone who struggles with their mental health and well-being wants to learn a specific exercise modality, it's important not to dismiss what they want to learn as not mindful enough or not capable of developing focus and openness.

Alternatively, any exercise or movement modality can also be done mindlessly, including traditionally mindful disciplines, like yoga or Tai Chi. I taught group yoga classes semi-regularly for years, and I learned to recognize the person who would sit at the back, ignore instructions, and always take the hardest variation of the pose, even when it wasn't, perhaps, the most appropriate choice. The nature of private sessions makes it easier for me to identify what the client connects with and choose words or tasks to redirect when I observe a client disconnecting (which happens, and isn't necessarily bad. What matters is that they are able to return to the present moment).

For the purposes of this chapter, I am defining gentle movement as movement that is done slowly, giving the client an opportunity to slow down and feel what is happening. I often refer to this as restorative movement, which clients understand means movement that is being performed with the intention of helping them tap into subtlety. While the research in this area primarily focuses on yoga, Tai Chi, and Pilates, there are underlying themes that most mindful movement modalities share. Once you understand these themes, you can apply the principles behind mindful movement in a variety of settings.

Yoga and Mental Health

Yoga has become a popular form of mindful movement in the United States and Europe. Yoga is a discipline and practice that originated in India. Most forms of yoga practiced in the United States are Hatha yoga, defined by researchers as including physical postures, breath work, and meditation (Uebelacker & Broughton, 2016).

Systematic reviews on yoga and anxiety are mixed regarding yoga's effectiveness. A review performed in 2016 (Cramer *et al.*, 2018) concluded that Hatha yoga might be beneficial as part of a comprehensive treatment program for individuals with anxiety, but there wasn't enough evidence to suggest that it was an effective standalone treatment.

More recent research found that a combination of meditation, yoga, and mindfulness led to a decrease in symptoms related to depression, anxiety, and stress in college-age students (Breedvelt *et al.*, 2019). Another study concluded that while mindful meditation programs may be effective for reducing psychological stress and improving well-being, so are other interventions such as behavioral therapy, relaxation, and exercise (Goyal *et al.*, 2014).

Something else to consider when thinking about whether yoga is an appropriate choice for someone with anxiety is the relationship between hypermobility and heightened interoceptive awareness. The fact that they are related means that sometimes a movement session devoted solely to developing interoceptive accuracy may not be appropriate for people with a heightened sense of interoception, at least not until they develop a baseline of strength. Beginning with interoception can feel overwhelming for some individuals and may not be as effective as other interventions for initially reducing symptoms related to anxiety.

The flip side to this is that people with a lot of natural flexibility tend to be "good" at the physical postures of yoga. We tend to like doing things we are naturally good at, so people with lots of flexibility might find themselves drawn to the yoga practice, only to miss out on the mental benefits they were hoping to achieve. Being "good" at the physical postures causes positive feelings because of that powerful hit of dopamine you are rewarded with when you successfully complete something. Unless the yoga is being taught in a strength-based way, it won't increase a sense of physical and emotional resilience, and if it is being taught in a strength-based way, it may still not be as effective at reducing anxiety initially, because most forms of yoga ask the practitioner to focus inward. This can backfire, causing the student to feel overwhelmed and worried about their internal state.

On the other hand, If the student isn't hypermobile and doesn't have heightened interoceptive awareness, yoga may be extremely effective at creating more PSNS/SNS balance.

A client I have been working with for a long time said to me recently, "When did you get into all of this breath work? It changed my life when you began teaching it to me. I no longer have to carry around Xanax just in case I have a panic attack." (Breath work is often taught in yoga classes. In fact, 6 of the 8 studies included in the review by Cramer *et al.* (2018) on Hatha yoga and anxiety had a breathing component.) Granted, breath work is a small part of this particular client's session, but it's an important part.

In contrast, I worked with another woman for a long time, who was hypermobile and didn't respond to breath work at all. It created more stress, as she tried to make sure she was doing it right and became concerned that she wasn't feeling it where she was supposed to. She had a lot of interoceptive awareness but not a lot of interoceptive accuracy, and her concern for what she was doing and how she was doing it eliminated the potential benefits. (I rerouted and moved more towards externally based instructions and tasks with her, which worked well, giving her a baseline of strength and more confidence.)

There are, of course, a number of benefits to yoga, including the fact that it is relatively affordable and readily accessible in many areas. Yoga can be practiced either in a class setting or at home, under the guidance of streaming videos or books (Uebelacker & Broughton, 2016), and there are yoga classes for a wide variety of conditions, making it feel more accessible than, say, CrossFit. (Not that accessible CrossFit doesn't exist. It's just that you are more likely to see a pre-natal yoga class or yoga geared towards special populations like individuals with cancer and multiple sclerosis (MS) than you are a similar CrossFit class.)

Researchers speculate that yoga might impact depression and anxiety in a variety of ways. Most forms of yoga direct attention in a non-judgmental way, which interrupts the default mode network and can have carry-over in everyday life. Being attentive to current experiences reminds people that feelings are transient in nature, shifting throughout the course of the day. Yoga may also regulate the ANS and decrease inflammation. Is it more effective than other mindful exercise programs? At this time, it's impossible to say, but that doesn't mean people who are interested in yoga for mental health benefits shouldn't be encouraged to try it.

Additionally, because mindfulness is associated with activation of several different brain regions, it may create more fluid connections between the executive control network (aka the paying attention network), the default mode network (the mind wandering network), and the salience network (the "I am aware I am daydreaming" network and/or the "Ooh! Look! A rainbow-tailed squirrel! I am going to observe my interest in this squirrel" network) (Doll et al., 2015).

The salience network is also the part of your brain that recognizes that your mind is wandering, which means it's working when you are practicing any sort of open monitoring. It's also involved in detecting and integrating things like sensory stimuli and emotional stimuli, which means it is involved in interoceptive processing (Ku et al., 2020).

Like all things, ideally there would be an interplay between these networks, creating a semblance of balance. Fluidity and flexibility between networks plays a role in creating a more mentally and emotionally adaptable human.

Though the number of randomized controlled trials on yoga and PTSD is sparse, the results appear promising. Yoga breathing led to a decrease in PTSD symptoms in individuals after the 2004 Asian tsunami (Descilo *et al.*, 2010). Yoga also led to a decrease in hyperarousal symptoms in women with PTSD (but symptoms also decreased in the control group, suggesting that self-monitoring may have played a role in reducing symptoms) (Mitchell *et al.*, 2014). As with clients with anxiety and depression, yoga should be considered if the client with PTSD is interested; if the client isn't interested, other forms of movement may lead to higher adherence.

Tai Chi and Mental Health

The studies performed so far on Tai Chi and mental health tend to have significant limitations. However, despite these limitations, the results show that Tai Chi interventions may be beneficial for improving psychological well-being in individuals with depression and anxiety. It also may improve general stress management and exercise self-efficacy (Wang *et al.*, 2014; Sharma & Haider, 2015; Yin & Dishman, 2014).

Tai Chi is a traditional Chinese martial art that combines deep diaphragmatic breathing and relaxation with fundamental postures, or positions, that flow seamlessly from one to another through slow, graceful movements (Yang *et al.*, 2015). As with yoga, there are many forms of Tai Chi, and the practice can range in intensity and duration. Also like yoga, the practice is relatively affordable and can be modified to suit most people. This may make it feel like a safe form of movement for individuals who are worried about injuring themselves.

Tai Chi has been shown to increase balance, aerobic capacity, muscular strength, and flexibility in older patients with chronic conditions (Zhang *et al.*, 2012). It appears to improve self-esteem and reduce mood disturbances; it may also improve self-efficacy in individuals with various diseases and across different populations (Wang *et al.*, 2010).

While Tai Chi has a long history dating back to its 15th-century origin, its modern form referred to here is a form of exercise that promotes physical and psychological well-being through balance, postural control, and movement coordination (Zhang *et al.*, 2012). It may lead to improvements in blood pressure, reduced fall risk for fall-prone older adults, and improved dynamic balance, making it a good exercise choice for those who want a gentle introduction to movement (Nguyen & Kruse, 2012).

Tai Chi may also be beneficial for individuals post trauma. When veterans with Gulf War illness, a chronic disorder whose symptoms include fatigue, sleep disturbances, psychological problems, and widespread pain, participated in a Tai Chi program, they slept better than veterans who stretched and did low-impact exercise (Reid *et al.*, 2019). (High sleep quality is associated with decreases in chronic pain and improved psychological outcomes.)

Regular Tai Chi significantly reduced stress, anxiety, and depression in community-dwelling patients with chronic conditions, and research suggests that Tai Chi may reduce chronic pain associated with osteoarthritis (*ibid.*).

One of the main differences between yoga and Tai Chi is the amount of stillness. Yoga is typically taught with an emphasis on finding stillness and staying in postures for a while before moving on to the next posture. Tai Chi is taught using slow, deliberate movements, moving slowly from one position to the next. Is one better than the other? No: sometimes, finding stillness is exactly what the person needs to find more physiological and emotional balance; sometimes, slowly moving from one position to the next with less of an emphasis on stillness is what someone needs. Using modalities or movements that encourage paying attention to the task at hand while moving slowly and thoughtfully can focus a person's attention, shifting the emphasis from the default mode network to the salience network or the executive control network. The simple act of moving slowly can create the illusion of time slowing down; it can also bring someone into the present moment in a way that re-establishes a sense of equanimity.

Nowadays, I don't teach yoga or Tai Chi, though I borrow from elements of both. I have clients who see me for the slower work, as a way to reset their nervous system and recreate the mind/body connection they feel they have lost. I have been told more than once it's like getting a massage, except no one actually touches you and the experience is more internal. Trying different modalities and taking the time to carve out a slower, thoughtful practice for yourself can make it easier to know what to recommend for clients or help you implement concepts when people need a different type of movement session. I am not suggesting that everyone becomes a yoga or Tai Chi teacher, but being able to incorporate short elements of mindful movement during a session can be hugely beneficial for some clients.

The Benefits of Group Settings

The following reasons have been suggested to explain why exercise benefits personal well-being (Chow & Tsang, 2007):

- *Cognitive behavioral hypothesis*: To paraphrase Reese Wither-spoon's character Elle from *Legally Blond*, exercise makes people happy. It generates positive thoughts and feelings, and overcoming challenging physical tasks causes feelings associated with accomplishment and increased self-efficacy. Basically, it makes you all warm and fuzzy inside.
- *Social interaction hypothesis*: Exercising with people is pleasurable, and since we are social animals, the shared experience improves mental health. You know the energy you feel when you are with your favorite people at a dinner party? Exercising with people can recreate that sensation.
- *Distraction*: Exercise is an opportunity to be distracted from everyday life worries, taking your mind off the things that are a source of stress and anxiety. It is difficult to think about when the water bill is due when you are trying to figure out how to bend your elbows so your legs will lift off the floor or trying to decide if you can actually lift the barbell off the ground with that many plates on it. Your brain is remarkably good at focusing when the challenge is high enough.
- *Cardiovascular fitness hypothesis*: As you become more aerobically fit, your mood improves. I am a perpetually happy person. My husband claims it's all the running and biking I do. He might be right.
- *Amine/endorphin theory*: Exercise stimulates the production of neurotransmitters that cause an increase in general well-being. What causes all of those warm fuzzy feelings I talked about just a moment ago? Neurotransmitters.

Exercising in a group or class setting taps into several of these theories. Group exercise settings may be particularly beneficial from a biopsychosocial perspective, because group exercise is a social activity that increases well-being. Simply being in a room with others elicits a shared experience, and when classes incorporate partner work or task-based activities that require the student to focus or provide an interesting challenge, the experience becomes meaningful on a deeper level. The shared experience creates a sense of belonging, an adaptive human need that amplifies emotions and creates connection (Jolly *et al.*, 2019). Shared experiences also increase the value on a personal level and are more likely to be remembered than solo experiences of the same thing (Min *et al.*, 2017). We will discuss partner work more in Chapter 6.

I have now discussed two common examples of mindful exercise— Tai Chi and yoga—but can other forms of exercise be mindful? How can mindful exercise be interspersed into a traditional exercise setting in a beneficial way?

A (Brief) History of Mindful Movement

Movement designed to unify the body and the mind was originally documented in ancient Greek culture in calisthenics, a philosophy that was practiced to facilitate self-empowerment and prepare individuals for rigorous athletic and military events. (Calisthenics is a Greek word that means strength and beauty.)

Early documentation of Western mind/body philosophies dates back to the late 18th century, when Swedish medical gymnastics teacher Pehr Henrik Ling developed an apparatus-free method to improve functional movement and prevent and heal human disease. Ling believed non-strenuous, rhythmical, functional movement was a way to manage and prevent musculoskeletal disorders, maintain a healthy body and mind, and enhance athletic performance (Hoffman & Gabel, 2015).

Around the same time, Friedrich Ludwig Jahn, a Prussian nationalist and exercise instructor, invented the standard equipment used in modern gymnastics, including the parallel bars, rings, and balance beam. He founded the Physical Culture Movement and, along with Ling, gained a following of enthusiasts for the holistic, non-competitive exercise systems. This changed in the late 19th century, when the gymnasium environment shifted towards more strenuous training, favoring bodybuilding methods and competitive gymnastics over the non-competitive approaches rooted in connecting the mind and the body.

What happened next was interesting and came to define what we think of today as mind/body exercise. Mind/body enthusiasts split off, opening independent schools where opinions could be expressed freely. There were six pioneers who emerged with similar exercise philosophies and practicing similar exercises: Checkley, Muller, Alexander, Randell, Pilates, and Morris.

Although all these people had an influence on the current state of mind/body disciplines, several didn't become household names. Checkley believed in movement that was non-competitive and equipment free, and didn't exhaust someone mentally or physically. Mueller was a Danish athlete who published the book *My System*, describing how the average person could increase mental and physical efficiency with 15 minutes of daily exercise. Randall was inspired by Ling's philosophy and believed exercise was a form of preventative medicine. She developed pre-natal training and post-natal training techniques to help stay strong mentally and physically before and after childbirth. Morris founded Margaret Morris Movement using natural dance moves to create a healthy mind and body. She emphasized the connection between breathing, stamina, range of motion, and posture as portals to health and vitality.

Only two of the six, Alexander and Pilates, went on to become well recognized in later years for their contributions to Western mind/body philosophies.

Frederick Matthias Alexander is best known for creating the Alexander Technique, a holistic movement technique that evolved from his work with stage artists and people with breathing trouble. He used mindful postures and movements to re-establish conscious control of movement and posture. He was against weightlifting and felt that working muscles in isolation wasn't healing. The Alexander Technique differs from other mind/body disciplines in that the development of nervous system control is emphasized first, before improvements in function. Other systems develop the nervous system after doing exercises in the "proper" manner. Of course, we know that it is impossible to develop just one aspect of the neuromuscular system. Fortunately, as our understanding of science has evolved, so has our understanding of how why different systems and methodologies work.

Joseph Hubertus Pilates is perhaps the most famous of these six individuals. He was born in Germany, and practiced wrestling and gymnastics as a child. He moved to Scotland as a young adult, becoming a fitness trainer for Scotland Yard, but during the outbreak of WWI in 1914 he was placed in an "alien camp" due to his nationality. While detained, he trained inmates and developed his method, Contrology. He was eventually moved to the Isle of Man, where he trained injured inmates. In order to make movement accessible for those who were injured, he connected springs to the hospital beds, which later evolved into modern Pilates equipment.

After WWI, Pilates moved back to Germany and began working with dancers. However, he didn't want the German army using his methods, so he moved to Manhattan, where he quickly gained popularity with dancers and celebrities. He believed corrective exercise was the only way to develop a strong, pain-free body. He advocated breathing and training outside in the sun. In the 34 exercises in the Contrology home routine, he purposefully left out standing exercises to eliminate undue strain on the heart and optimize position of the viscera. (Fortunately, we now know standing isn't bad for the heart, and the viscera are supported in a variety of positions.)

The Emergence of Mind/Body Techniques in Psychotherapy

As the mind/body movement was gaining momentum and differentiating itself from fitness in the West, body psychotherapy, a form of therapy that explores what's happening in the body as a way to more deeply understand emotions and feeling states, was emerging in psychotherapy. Wilhelm Reich was a student of Freud's. He wrote the treatise *Character Analysis* in 1933 and is considered the pioneer of body psychotherapy. He felt that neurotic symptoms were not just rooted in thoughts or feelings, but also contained physiological and physical aspects. Body and mind, he realized, were intimately connected, and habitual physical tensions, he believed, were both protective and restrictive, preventing the experience of pleasure and joy.

His work influenced many who went on to champion the connection between the mind and the body, including Jack Rosenberg, founder of Gestalt Body Psychotherapy, and Ron Kurtz, founder of the Hakomi Method. A characteristic inherent in all forms of body psychotherapy is the belief that the self is embodied—that emotions are felt and experienced in and through the body (Young, 2010).

In the mid-20th century, Eugene Gendlin, a student of psychotherapist Carl Rogers, identified a way of knowing though attentiveness to the body and its wisdom. He coined the term "felt sense"; the ability to tune in to the felt sense and to be with the experience is called focusing (Watson, 2013; Schoeller & Dunaetz, 2018). His work is a way to experience emotion more implicitly and emphasizes the ability to tune in to the body and what it's saying.

Somatics

Somatics was described by Thomas Hanna as the study and practices associated with the discovery and development of the body and its experiences (Mullan, 2012). These practices invite exploration through attention to movement and perception.

Hanna studied with Moshé Feldenkrais and went on to develop his own somatic method, Hanna Somatics. Feldenkrais is often considered a pioneer in the field of somatics. He developed a self-education system that focuses on developing bodily awareness through movement. Feldenkrais's work is based on a variety of disciplines, including physics, anatomy, neuroscience, learning theories, Judo and other martial arts, and mind/body practices (Smyth, 2016). The emphasis on bodily self-awareness during Awareness Through Movement lessons (ATMs) was considered by Gendlin to be more subtle and fleeting, like a mood. The ability to find yourself in that moment is the goal of both Feldenkrais ATM and focusing exercises, the main difference being that the sense of self is found during Feldenkrais ATMs through movement, while focusing uses directed attention and does not necessarily include movement.

Elsa Gindler, who spent her entire life in Berlin, is often considered the grandmother of somatic psychology and body psychotherapy. Originally a student of Harmonische Gymnastik ("Harmonic Gymnastics" in English), she founded a teacher training school in 1917. Gymnastik didn't refer to the sport of gymnastics; rather, it was a movement education and somatic awareness system, similar to the early gymnastics programs taught by Ling. Gindler eventually left Harmonische Gymnastik, feeling it was too narrow in its focus (Mullan, 2017). Her teachings, which she never named, encouraged people to explore and develop individually and independently. It was a practice uniting mind, body, and spirit that influenced the teachings of others (Geuter *et al.*, 2010).

Rudolf Laban, a Hungarian man born in 1879 to a military family, is considered the father of European modern dance. His method, the Laban Movement Analysis system, was originally developed through the context of dance using observation and analysis of movement based on knowledge of somatics and embodiment. Its benefits have been recognized as being far-reaching, and it has influenced practices in factory labor, robotics, and therapy (Bernardet *et al.*, 2019).

Bonnie Bainbridge Cohen, an occupational therapist who also studied dance, developed a system called Body-Mind Centering to facilitate healing. It utilizes experimental learning rather than a prescribed set of exercises, to explore and encourage improvised movement. She continues to teach, and her work influences many somatic therapists.

The list of individuals above outlines a few of the people and systems who influence many of the mind/body practices that are performed today but is by no means exhaustive. There are many more who have influenced these fields, but I hope the breadth and cross-pollination of ideas serves as a reminder that there are many ways to achieve the same outcome, as long as basic principles are followed. There are basic principles many of these disciplines have in common, which we will discuss next. Before we move on, reflect for a moment on the last time you participated in a mind/body exercise modality that you found particularly effective. Where was the attention focused? What aspect of the experience resonated with you? Did you notice a shift in your mood after the class or session?

Now imagine that someone with a very different personality than yours took the same class. Do you think they would feel the same way when class ended? If you are struggling to understand what I mean, imagine this: Sue, an intelligent woman with low energy who likes moving slowly and focusing on being in the present moment takes a restorative yoga class and afterwards feels amazing. Brian, an intelligent man with high energy who dislikes sitting still and prefers to focus on what's next takes the same restorative yoga class and dislikes it intensely, not feeling any calmer when class is over. Whose experience is "right"?

Both of their experiences and responses are completely valid. It's okay for Brian to not find restorative yoga relaxing, just like it's okay for Sue to find restorative yoga works really well to downregulate her nervous system. Restorative yoga, then, becomes a viable option as a mind/body modality for Sue that may help with her mental well-being, while for Brian, if his goal is to find a slower, mindful modality, he may need to try a few more things before he discovers the one that works.

I am like Brian. I have a lot of energy, I am a doer, I like to move, and I find stillness as a form of meditation challenging, unless it's the three minutes I carve out daily after running and performing my movement practice to focus on my breath. I spent four years doing weekly Feldenkrais lessons, which, while effective, were always performed after running and I rarely made it through more than 40 minutes of the lesson. Restorative yoga feels anything but restorative, which is why my ten-year-long yoga practice consisted of Ashtanga, a dynamic form of yoga that's performed in a sequenced manner, staying in most positions for five breaths before moving to the next. This, it turns out, wasn't restorative either, and it wasn't until I began regularly implementing the principles outlined later in this chapter that I was able to truly tap into a movement practice that hones a mind/body connection that works for me.

This isn't to say I didn't need to find ways to slow down. I absolutely did, and when I learned how to move slowly, breathe, center, and ground, I became less anxious and more embodied. People who already move regularly and are strong and aerobically fit can often benefit hugely from finding softness and more subtlety, just like people who are inactive can experience huge mental benefits from gaining strength and endurance.

Part of the practitioner's responsibility is to find ways to access embodiment in clients for whom exercise means hard and fast. These are the clients who don't need to be encouraged to exercise, because they do it daily, and who have a difficult time slowing down to feel.

Earlier chapters have shown that exercise is beneficial for mental health. A large study that surveyed the exercise habits and mental health status of 1.2 million people over the age of 18 found that physical activity was significantly and meaningfully associated with feeling better mentally (Chekroud et al., 2018). The magic amount of exercise seemed to be 45 minutes of vigorous exercise three to five times per week. More exercise wasn't necessarily better; in fact, people who exercised for more than 90 minutes a session had a slight decrease in mental health, and exercising for more than three hours per session was associated with worse mental health than not exercising at all.

Mindful exercise, which was defined as yoga and Tai Chi, correlated with a statistically significant improvement in people's mental health when they were compared with non-exercising individuals (*ibid.*).

This is consistent with what research shows for people who compulsively exercise. Negative running addiction was defined in 1982 by researchers Jo Hailey and Leisa Bailey, who created the Negative Addiction Scale. (Researcher William Glasser posited that running was a positive addiction in the 1970s; it wasn't until a few years later that experts realized that there were potentially harmful effects of compulsive exercise.) Since then, a growing body of research suggests that exercise and sport can be consistent with compulsive behavior that has negative consequences, including injuries and links to eating and affective disorders (Lichtenstein *et al.*, 2017).

In one particularly disturbing study, researchers found a strong association between subjects with bulimia nervosa who also over-exercised and suicidal behaviors. The researchers speculated that the decrease in anxiety-related body sensations may increase the risk for suicidal behavior. The lack of pain sensitivity that occurs in individuals who become habituated to chronic overuse injuries may lead to an increase in a person's capability for self-harm (Smith *et al.*, 2018).

What's particularly difficult about this is that the very thing that makes exercise extremely beneficial for many people (the decrease in fear about bodily sensations) may be detrimental in certain groups.

Fortunately, it does appear that mind/body movement may be beneficial in subjects with eating disorders who also over-exercise. A small study found that a yoga intervention combined with outpatient eating disorder treatment led to a significant decrease in anxiety, depression, and body image disturbance (*ibid.*). High levels of yoga practice may promote body awareness and appreciation while decreasing self-objectification and promoting embodiment (Neumark-Sztainer, 2013).

Individuals with anorexia nervosa may benefit from Qigong, a mind/body discipline from which Tai Chi originates. A very small study (16 adolescent females) concluded that Qigong was an interesting therapeutic tool when combined with psychotherapy in contributing to the recovery process in individuals with anorexia nervosa. Its emphasis on slow movements, interoceptive awareness, and self-massage reduced the sense of competition and gave individuals an opportunity to enhance their sense of self. This may reduce body-related anxiety, improve body acceptance, and promote nutrition adherence (Gueguen *et al.*, 2017).

Mindful Movement Principle I: Breath

Now that you understand the most commonly studied forms of mindful movement and how they may contribute to mental well-being, let's focus on what these modalities have in common.

There are four basic principles of mindful movement that are consistent across most of the disciplines highlighted above. How these principles are introduced varies across the modalities, but understanding the basic components means you can apply these concepts to any movement practice to promote mindful movement. This will help your clients re-establish connection with their bodies and, hopefully, will bring benefits to other areas of their lives.

The first principle of mindful movement is breathing. Breath work or awareness is interesting. It can make people with a heightened interoceptive awareness feel dizzy, more anxious, or mildly claustrophobic if it's introduced too soon or in a way that doesn't resonate with the client. Instead of downregulating the SNS, it can activate the SNS, foiling your well-intentioned plan to help your client feel more relaxed and connected.

Fortunately, there are ways to significantly reduce the chances of this happening. Before we get into ways to incorporate breathing, I will examine why breathing is considered such an integral part of mindful movement and how it affects the PSNS.

TRY THIS: Come into a comfortable position. If you are seated on the floor, feel your sitting bones against the floor. If you are seated on the chair, feel your sitting bones on the chair and your feet on the floor.

Take a moment to observe how you feel. This is purposefully vague and may refer to how you feel physically or emotionally. Just notice what draws your attention.

Set a timer for two minutes. Observe your breath, watching the inhale and exhale. Don't change the breath, simply watch it, noticing where it goes and what you feel when it leaves.

When the timer goes off, take another moment to observe how you feel. Do you feel different?

This particular exercise highlights how fleeting feeling can be. Often, people will feel a subtle shift after two minutes, which is a valuable reminder that how we are experiencing each moment is temporary.

The time is purposefully short, and if you include an exercise like this at the end of a movement or exercise session, it can make it easier for people who don't like to "waste" time meditating to take a moment to slow down and pause. Not trying to change the breath gives people who may be sensitive to breath work an entry point, allowing them to check in with how their breath moves through their bodies. It's not unusual for the breathing to quiet down and the breath to shift subtly when the time is finished.

The Anatomy of the Breath

The diaphragm is the muscle associated with inhalation and exhalation. The lungs are passive, responding to the pressure changes caused by the diaphragm and intercostal muscles as they contract and relax. These muscle movements cause air to either enter the lungs or be expelled from the lungs (Molnar & Gair, 2015).

The diaphragm is innervated by the phrenic nerve, which originates from the cervical spine. An easy mnemonic for the innervation of the diaphragm is "C3, 4, 5, keep the diaphragm alive." The phrenic nerve provides motor and sensory information to the diaphragm, as well as sympathetic nerve fibers. Can you remember which nerve supplies parasympathetic nerve fibers to the diaphragm? (Clue: it's also called the wandering nerve.)

If you came up with cranial nerve X, the vagus nerve, you are correct (Bordoni *et al.*, 2018). Remember, when vagus tone is high, or the vagus nerve is activated, the PSNS is in high gear, resting and digesting. How would you expect the breathing to be during this state? It would be slower, more relaxed, and through the nose, with fewer accessory muscles involved. Breathing through the nose modulates limbic oscillations, which means it helps control activity in the limbic part of the brain (Zelano *et al.*, 2016). The limbic system is the part of the brain controlled in fear response, and nasal breathing appears to specifically modulate activity in the amygdala and hippocampus. Nasal breathing, then, may impact emotional well-being by regulating the part of the brain associated with detecting fear.

What happens when breathing is being driven by the SNS? The breath will be shorter, more rapid, and shallower. The accessory muscles of inspiration will be more active, since the breath will be more active. These muscles include the trapezius, pectoralis major, pectoralis minor, and sternocleidomastoid (Oliver & Ashurst, 2018). It should come as no surprise that one of the physical manifestations of symptoms associated with anxiety and depression is neck pain (Blozik *et al.*, 2009).

The diaphragm is a skeletal muscle that concentrically contracts during inhalation. The exhale leads to a passive recoil, unless there is conscious effort to slow down the exhale or resistance is applied to strengthen the diaphragm eccentrically (this can be done by breathing into a balloon or a straw). Though the contraction and relaxation of the diaphragm is primarily done unconsciously, there are phrenic motor neurons that can be activated consciously, giving you (partial) control over how you breathe (Fogarty *et al.*, 2018).

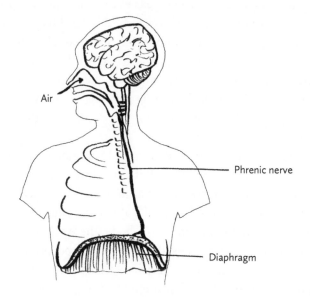

DIAPHRAGM AND PHRENIC NERVE

A review concluded that slow breathing techniques were effective for increasing heart rate variability by activating PSNS activity (Zaccaro *et al.*, 2018). It found that slow breathing also improved psychological markers by improving comfort and relaxation and decreasing arousal, anxiety, depression, and anger.

Breathing is an important aspect of our sense of safety. It regulates mood; conversely, mood can alter breathing. Drawing attention to the breath occasionally and incorporating breath work through specific positions or movements can help clients become aware of their own breathing habits.

It probably won't be a surprise that improving someone's sense of safety can alter their breathing patterns. For instance, if you are working with someone with symptomatic benign joint hypermobility, aka JHS, breath work may not be a good choice, particularly initially. JHS is linked to increased interoceptive awareness, which is also linked to higher anxiety, higher pain perception, and decreased proprioception (Bulbena-Cabre & Bulbena, 2018). Interestingly, people who are hypermobile also appear to have higher amygdala volume than people without hypermobility, possibly because people with hypermobility have heightened susceptibility to the threat of pain and/or disturbances in autonomic control (Eccles *et al.*, 2012).

JHS is also correlated with decreased proprioception, specifically lower-limb joint position sense, compared with those without JHS (Smith *et al.*, 2013). Decreased joint position sense would (hypothetically) reduce an individual's sense of personal safety—it feels more secure to know where the limbs are in relation to the environment. This uncertainty in limb position alters breathing patterns, so one way to change breathing patterns is by improving proprioception and stability through a targeted strength program.

I have witnessed this with symptomatic hypermobile clients. Breath work increases anxiety due to the heightened interoceptive awareness; giving them a strength intervention that connects them with their physical bodies and creates a sense of stability alters breathing in a visible way.

All of these systems (the brain, the body, the ANS) work together. Altering one will affect the others. If you work with people in an individualized setting, the more you can learn to recognize what clients need through their movements and through listening, the better equipped you will be to offer an intervention that positively impacts them, mentally and physically.

Putting Breath into Practice

Some ideas for introducing breath work with clients are given below. The ideas are relatively simple, a way to introduce the concept. I will cover more concentrated, positional breath work in Chapter 7 when I discuss practical applications.

Does the client periodically hold their breath? If so, it's important for you, the practitioner, to notice. Here are some questions you can ask yourself:

- When does the client tend to hold their breath?
- Are they holding their breath to create spinal stability?
- If they are using it to create a sense of spinal stability, what can you do to give them a greater sense of spinal stability?
- When the client begins to breathe again, do they mouth breathe or nose breathe?

In my experience, people hold their breath for one (or both) of the following two reasons:

- It's a learned habit they do under stressful situations.
- They don't have a sense of strength/stability in their spine.

Does the person hold their breath when you are asking them to balance or learn something new? If so, it's likely a response to stress (remember: breathing through the nose regulates limbic oscillations). Not breathing at all will impact the emotional response to the new/stressful situation. A simple intervention might be to ask the client, "Are you breathing?" This draws their awareness to their breath and reminds them to breathe without telling them *how* to breathe.

Or, does the person hold their breath when you ask them to lift something, change positions, or do anything resembling abdominal work? If so, breath holding may be a learned behavior to create a sense of spinal stability. While asking the person to breathe may improve awareness, it won't address the underlying problem of feeling unstable.

Intra-abdominal pressure (IAP) is defined as:

> The steady-state pressure that occurs within the abdominal cavity that results from the interaction between the abdominal wall and the viscera. The breathing cycle causes oscillations in IAP based on phase of respiration and abdominal wall resistance. (Milanesi & Caregnato, 2016)

IAP increases during static and dynamic lifting tasks. A common strategy when effort is required is to inhale, pause, exhale. The pause has been used in research settings to produce higher peak IAP than other forms of breath control. This suggests that breath holding is an effective strategy when lifting something heavy (Hagins *et al.*, 2004). However, if this becomes the strategy for low-threshold activities, like lifting a foam roller or transitioning from a sitting to a standing position, this is no longer efficient. You can think of it as an overreaction to tasks that require low amounts of effort. Introducing proper regressions and reminding the person to breathe during the low-level regressions creates a safe situation with minimal threat. This allows the client to explore other strategies for spinal stabilization.

One way to use breathing during a movement session is to use breathing as isometric pauses. If you use isometric pauses to develop strength and mobility in specific positions, ask the person you are working with to hold the position for two to four breaths rather that for a specific amount of time. Not only does this distract the client from the (likely) discomfort of the isometric contraction, it also gives them a short moment to focus on breathing.

You can also introduce breathing as a way to cool down. At the end of a workout or movement session, ask the client to watch their breath while in a comfortable position. I often use a supine position with the knees bent and the feet flat on the floor, but you could use whatever position the client finds comfortable, whether that's legs up the wall, legs long, lying down on a foam roller, knees on a foam roller, sitting, standing, prone...there is no "right" position for breathing.

I usually introduce it like this: "As you inhale, watch your breath as it enters your nose and travels throughout your body. As you exhale, observe the path the breath takes as it moves out. Spend the next few breaths watching your breath, observing its journey."

I find that people are often more receptive to observing and focusing on the breath when it is used as a cool-down after they have moved their bodies. Movement systems that instruct every breath with every movement take away from the body's intelligence and self-organization. We know that breathing (or not breathing) can be used to elicit several physical experiences, such as increasing spinal stiffness, feeling more sensation in the lower abdominals, improving proprioception, and creating more mobility through the middle back and/or thoracic spine. However, just like every movement doesn't need to emphasize strength or subtlety, not every movement needs to emphasize breath. Introduce breath work gradually, just like you would introduce the progressions to a strength exercise gradually, until eventually the diaphragm becomes stronger, the breath becomes calmer, and the client can use the breath as one way to enhance their practice.

Mindful Movement Principle II: Grounding

The second aspect to a mindful movement practice is grounding. Grounding can mean a couple of different things, depending on how it is being utilized. In a research setting, the term "grounded cognition" is sometimes used interchangeably with "embodied cognition" to represent how we process the environment around us. Proponents of grounded cognition think information processing is dependent on information from both the sensory and motor aspects of the nervous system. How we interpret that information affects our ability to retrieve and apply information appropriately (Hayes & Kraemer, 2017).

For instance, if you practice parkour regularly, when you see a rail, the area of your brain that is activated during balance and motor control may light up as you ponder different ways to balance on the rail off the ground.

If, on the other hand, you have never thought about standing or crawling on a rail, the rail represents something different—maybe a way to define space or something to hold on to while you climb stairs.

Our view of the world is shaped by our experiences, which is, perhaps, why grounding in a psychological sense is often loosely defined as using your senses to connect your mind and body. Let's say you are having a rough day, your brain is going a million miles a minute, and you are having a hard time focusing. If you look around the room until your eyes rest on something interesting, and you let your eyes settle on the interesting object, you are using your visual sense to ground you to something that is actually in the here and now.

The grounding that is commonly referenced in a movement setting is similar, though it relates more to using proprioceptive and kinesthetic awareness to root you in the present moment. There is a small body of research that explores the effects of grounding on the body. Another term for this is "earthing," and it refers to bringing the body in contact with the earth—the actual earth—like walking barefoot on trails or on the beach (Chevalier, 2015). The reasons grounding works in this context may have more to do with the earth's electrons than the afferent nervous system, but I hope you will see, through the explanation offered below, how feeling the ground beneath you, even in an indoor setting, can integrate different senses and is an important aspect to mindful movement practices (Chevalier et al., 2012).

Grounding and Exteroception

A brief recap on exteroception: this is how you process the input you receive from your external environment; "exteroceptive awareness" specifically refers to the implicit knowledge someone has of their body and how it relates to space and movement based on the integration of exteroceptive signals. Senses related to exteroception are vision, touch, proprioception, smell, and hearing. Another term for exteroceptive awareness is "body schema" (Valenzuela-Moguillansky *et al.*, 2017).

The small studies on grounding that exist suggest that practicing grounding may be associated with reductions in pain and improvements in mood and physical function (Chevalier *et al.* 2019; Oschman *et al.*, 2015).

When you have a tangible representation of your contact with the ground, your body image—which is fluid and based on a number of factors, including mental and physical states—becomes, for lack of a better word, more rooted in the present moment. The result is a sense of body ownership that occurs because of our ability to integrate information from multiple senses (Stein *et al.*, 2014).

Pop quiz: Which two senses can easily be focused on when working on grounding and sensory input with clients?

Answer: Vision and the sense of touch as it relates to proprioception.

The ability to take in visual information regarding the surrounding environment enables us to do things like plan what we need to do in order to accurately reach for an object (Sarlegna & Sainburg, 2009). Vision is also critical for our ability to maintain balance. It works with proprioception and the vestibular system to reduce postural sway and enables us to recover from perturbations (Hansson *et al.*, 2010). One way to ground, then, is to ask clients to scan the room, noticing what's around them, and allow their eyes to settle on something comfortable. Ask them to keep their eyes on the object as they perform a specific task or skill.

Another way to use vision to ground someone is to have the client perform target-based tasks. I sometimes use the following exercise when I can tell clients are having a difficult time being present. It calms them down and helps them focus by using a variety of senses, including vision.

EXERCISE: REACHING FOR BLOCKS

Create a geometrical shape with five to eight blocks. Stand in the middle of the blocks. Keep your left leg planted as you reach your right foot to touch one of the blocks. Return your leg to the starting position. Repeat, touching each block gently with the right foot, and then switch legs.

Your vision and proprioception are what allow you to plan how you are going to reach for the block and set your foot back down. The reaching motion requires balance, but because your attention is distracted (the focus is on touching the block with the foot, not on how you are going to balance), the movement will be performed in an automatic, more fluid way than if you were thinking about how you were going to stay balanced while you reached your leg in different directions.

The same exercise can be performed standing on one leg or walking across a balance beam. The point is to have an actual object to reach for while performing a low-level balance task (which, of course, is relative, so pick the appropriate exercise for the client).

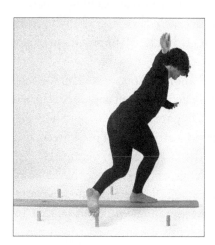
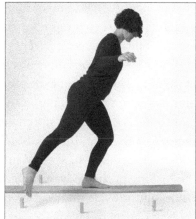

Grounding, Proprioception, and Kinesthetic Awareness

Proprioception plays a critical role in the ability to learn how to perform new movement skills (De Santis *et al.*, 2015). If proprioception is highly developed, motor learning happens more easily; when proprioception is impaired, motor learning happens more slowly. Developing proprioception makes learning new movement skills easier and adds more nuanced information to the brain about the body's position in space and its available options for movement.

Proprioception refers to the sensation that arises from the sensory, or afferent, neurons that are part of the motor nervous system feedback loop. Proprioceptors are located in muscle, tendon, joints, and skin. These neurons provide information regarding limb position and movement, tension and force, sense of effort, and sense of balance to the CNS (Proske & Gandevia, 2012).

"Kinesthesia" was a term first introduced by Bastian in 1888 (Proske & Gandevia, 2009). It refers to the conscious sensations of limb position and movement, and though it is an aspect of proprioception, it is generally accepted that proprioception, like neuroception, is an unconscious process: the ability to respond appropriately to a perturbation in a way that minimizes risk of injury and allows you to regain balance, or to avoid stepping in a pothole by using an unusual, but appropriate, step. When I refer to consciously grounding a hand or foot, this grounding increases kinesthesia, which, in turn, will improve an individual's overall proprioceptive sense (Aman et al., 2015). It's a bit like teaching someone how to identify the sound of middle C on a piano—the ability to hear middle C doesn't guarantee perfect pitch, but it will improve a person's overall ability to detect different pitches.

There are over 100 cutaneous mechanoreceptors located on the sole of the foot. These afferent receptors are an important source of sensory information for maintaining balance. They are sensitive to both how the foot contacts the ground and changes in distribution of pressure across the sole of the foot. Information in the Golgi tendon organs (GTOs) (located in tendons of skeletal muscle) gives the CNS feedback about the loading of the body, while muscle spindles around the knee and ankle joint provide information about joint angle position relative to the trunk. All of this feedback creates a sense of stability and determines how we use our lower limbs. Thus, the more we are in contact with the feet through our ability to sense them and how they interact with the floor, the more movement options we will have and the more secure we will feel (Kennedy & Inglis, 2002).

This works on two different levels. Remember in Chapter 4 how I discussed balance and its potential role in anxiety? Teaching someone how to feel their feet will likely improve balance. Improving balance may downregulate the SNS, making the individual feel less anxious and more calm.

When you ask someone to sense how their feet are connecting to the ground, that conscious awareness enhances proprioception and adds extra richness to how they feel and experience that specific moment.

Being able to feel the different aspects of the hand against the floor works similarly. Like the foot, the hand is sensory rich. The fingertips are particularly receptive to touch. The palm of the hand is composed of a special type of skin that's particularly sensitive to texture and how different objects feel.

Research also suggests that stimulating the nerves of the hands and the wrist causes a reflexive firing of the muscles in the trapezius and the shoulder (which shouldn't be all that surprising, since loading any body part requires force to be dispersed). When you place weight on the hand, the muscles of the upper extremity will share the load, and when you reach for an object, the muscles in the upper extremity support the change in position (Alexander & Harrison, 2003). Reaching the hand towards the floor, then, serves as a way to allow the hand to feel, concretely, its location in space and provides valuable information about the position of the joints that support the hand up into the shoulder.

HAND AND TOUCH

EXERCISE: GROUNDING THE FEET

Come into a standing position with your shoes off and your feet flat on the floor. Begin gently rocking from your heels to the front of the feet. The heels may lift as you rock forward and the front of the feet might lift as you rock back. Do this eight to ten times.

When you stop rocking, feel the support of the ground beneath your feet. Begin to sense the center of the heels against the floor. See if you can feel the balls of the big toes and the balls of the pinkie toes against the floor as well. Imagine that there are lines connecting the center of the heels to the big-toe balls of the foot and the pinkie-toe balls of the foot.

As you imagine this triangular platform of your foot against the floor, place your hands on the top of your thighs. Slide the hands down the thighs towards your knees. Allow the heels to come off the ground as you slide your hands towards your knees, and allow them to come back to the floor as you slide your hands away from the knees. Do this four to six times.

Find a position where your knees feel soft and you feel supported fully by the triangles of your feet. How does that feel?

EXERCISE: GROUNDING THE HANDS

Come into a quadruped position with your knees under your hips and your hands under your shoulders. Feel the weight of the hands against the floor. Bend your elbows or set your hands further forward if you are unable to place your palms flat against the floor.

Gently rock your torso backward, away from your hands, and forward, towards your hands, eight to ten times. Feel the pressure of your hands against the floor as you rock. Observe how the pressure of the floor under your hands changes as you move forward and backward.

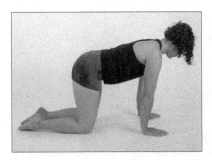 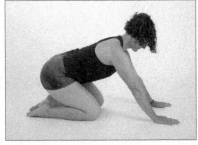

Pause in a position that feels, for lack of a better word, centered. Imagine that there is a line pressing the center of the palms into the floor. Think about pressure evenly distributing across your fingertips, from your thumb to your pinkie finger.

Bend your elbows and straighten them four to six times, seeing if you can maintain the contact of the center heels of the palms and the fingertips against the floor.

Pause in a position where it feels like your hands are able to easily support the arms. How does that feel?

If you lack the ability to ground the heel of the foot or the heel of the hand, you will receive less information about where your hand or foot is in relation to the floor. This impacts your ability to accurately perceive where your arms and legs are in relation to the ground and torso. Introducing gentle mobility exercises can make your entire system feel more safe and confident that you can move and interact with gravity in a non-harmful way.

Mindful Movement Principle III: Centering

Your center of mass is (probably) located slightly below your belly button at the level of the second sacral vertebrae. Center of mass is the central point on the human body; maintaining a center of mass within a base of support is essential for maintaining balance (An & Woo, 2017). Balance, remember, is associated with a sense of security; lack of balance is associated with anxiety.

Your base of support varies depending on what you are doing. It is the area beneath you, including the part of the body (or object) that makes contact with the ground. If you are standing with your feet evenly spaced, your base of support is your legs and your feet; balancing your center of mass over the legs and between the feet will provide a stable position.

If you stand on one leg, the base of support has shifted; your center of mass needs to be over the standing leg to maintain balance. The same thing happens when you take one hand to the floor, you stagger the feet, or you take both hands to the floor and the feet off the floor. The base of support changes, so the location of the center of mass changes to create balance.

Things get more complicated if you have an object beneath you. For instance, if you are riding a bicycle, your base of support is the two wheels. The center of mass becomes more complex because you have to take into account the center of mass of you—the human—plus the center of mass of the bicycle. This determines where, exactly, the center of mass is actually located and it's that point that needs to be centered over the two wheels to create balance.

Your center of mass moves when you move; where it moves and how much it moves is a determining factor in your ability to recover from a perturbation and maintain stability (Konig Ignasiak et al., 2019). If you are disconnected from your center of mass because you lack basic strength or stability, or because you don't occasionally utilize positions that require you to find your center, you won't feel stable. There will be a shift in how you use your body and your ability to feel stable. This reduces your proprioceptive accuracy and your ability to predict and recover from outside forces. Basically, it's harder for you to recover from being knocked over.

Orienting is a mental function that gives you a solid perception of your relationship to space, time, and people. It's a fundamental cognitive function that is related to several different processes and is intimately related to behavior (Peer et al., 2015). The ability to orient in space is dependent on where you perceive your sense of center to be, where your center of mass is located, and how it relates to the objects (and people) around you.

Your sense of center of mass can be influenced by things like hand dominance, foot dominance, and eye dominance (Zouhal et al., 2018). When you walk, the center of mass moves outside the base of support whenever the weight shifts from one leg to the other; a number of factors, including how you place the foot on the ground and the rotation of the pelvis, help you maintain a sense of stability while moving across the ground (Bruijn & van Dieen, 2018).

Your ability to accurately feel where your center of mass is located makes it less scary to move away from a stable balanced point. If, for instance, your sense of center is over your right foot when you are in a quiet standing position and someone pushes your left shoulder to the right, do you think it will be easy or difficult to maintain your balance? It will be difficult, because your sense of center is already over your right foot; a perturbation that pushes you further to the right leaves you with very few options, making it difficult to recover.

If, however, someone pushes your right shoulder to the left, your chances of success will be higher. Your brain will perceive a stable place to return to and it will feel like you could be pushed further to the left before being thrown off balance.

When your perception of your center of mass is more accurate, your brain will organize your extremities differently, in a more balanced way, while you are standing or sitting. You will feel more stable and your ability to move efficiently will increase because you will feel like you have a stable place to which to return.

This doesn't mean that you should strive for an ideal posture or that there is a specific way to sit or stand. It simply means that during a mindful movement practice, you can begin to explore your perception of center and your accuracy related to your perception. Mindful movement practices are also a great time to assess what it feels like to move away from center and return to center.

EXERCISE: FINDING CENTER IN STANDING

Begin in a comfortable standing position. Observe the sensation of your feet against the ground. Where does your weight settle? In the heels? In the middle of the foot? In the front of the foot? To the left? To the right?

Shift your hips back. Shift them forward. Go back and forth six to eight times.

Pause. Shift the weight to the left (you might imagine that you are shifting your belly button to the left). Shift the weight to the right. Go back and forth six to eight times.

Pause. Observe the weight in your feet. Does the weight feel more balanced?

EXERCISE: FINDING CENTER IN SEATED

Come into a comfortable seated position, either on the floor or in a chair. Observe the sensation of your sitting bones against the floor or chair.

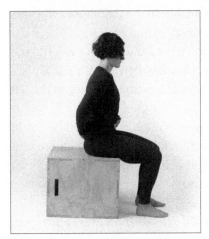 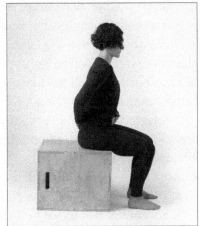

Rest your hands slightly below your belly button. Your eyes should be looking out so they are even with the horizon.

Begin gently rocking in front of your sitting bones and behind your sitting bones. Feel what happens to your belly beneath your hands as you rock forward and back.

Do this eight to ten times, moving slowly and sensing the change in position.

After your last time, rest in a place that feels centered. Imagine a line traveling from the center of your hands up to the breastbone and to the nose. Is the line straight?

EXERCISE: FINDING CENTER IN SUPINE

Lie on your back with your knees bent and your feet flat on the floor. Place one hand on your stomach, just below your belly button, and one hand on your chest. Imagine that there is a line traveling right down the center of you, connecting the two hands.

Pick your feet up off the floor one at a time so the knees are over the hips and the feet are in line with the knees. Rotate your torso to the right so both hands move at the same time. Don't go so far that you collapse over to the right side; just rotate enough that you can feel the rotation.

Return to center and rotate your torso to the left, maintaining a connection with the hands. Go back and forth between the two positions six to eight times.

Return to center and lower your feet back to the floor. Take a moment to relax and feel the imaginary line connecting your two hands. Is it any more clear?

EXERCISE: FINDING CENTER IN QUADRUPED

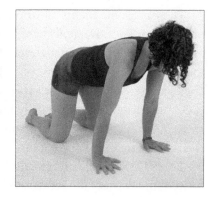

Come into a quadruped position, with your hands under your shoulders and your knees under your hips. Imagine the line connecting the center of your chest to the area just below your belly button. Is it straight?

Shift the imaginary line to the right and then shift it to the left. Continue shifting it from side to side six to eight times. When you finish, pause in the middle and reimagine the line. Is it more clear?

These exercises are a way to check in with your perception of center. They give you an opportunity to observe what you experience and contrast what you feel before and after a movement intervention, cultivating observation without judgment, the ability to focus attention, and listening.

Mindful Movement Principle IV: Listening

The final aspect of a mindful movement practice is listening. "Listening" simply refers to the ability to observe your experience in a nonjudgmental way. Another term for this is "open monitoring," which is also commonly referred to as mindfulness.

One of the keys to being mindful is observing. It can be easier to observe movement when you slow down; when you move fast, sometimes you miss the ability to observe fully. Slowing down movements and observing can help you ascertain sticking points, where you are losing coordination, and where you could be smoother and stronger.

Moving quickly allows you to move without overthinking. The observation that occurs when you move quickly happens after the movement is done. It becomes a reflection on the experience rather than a reflection in the experience.

Moving slowly is often thought of as a precursor to moving quickly—the more control you have when moving slowly, the more confident you will feel when moving quickly.

There are some clients for whom moving slowly is their jam. It's their favorite way to move, and these individuals should be encouraged to move quickly on occasion to develop power and confidence at different speeds. For many people, however, moving slowly is difficult, particularly if they don't want to feel or experience their physical selves. Moving slowly and listening can actually feel frustrating and/or scary. Asking these individuals to slow down and pause occasionally can help with their ability to reflect and listen.

These basic tenets of a mindful movement practice can be implemented in a variety of settings. While there are definitely people for whom a separate movement practice devoted entirely to mindful movement may be beneficial, for others, who may not have the time or interest, gently integrating these concepts throughout a session can make a huge difference to their ability to listen and feel.

The research on mindful movement, trauma, and depression consistently demonstrates a variety of potential benefits. People experience a shift in mood, a decrease in arousal, and an improved connection with the physical body. Paying attention to the individual in front of you and observing how they respond to your instructions and what piques their curiosity is the topic of the next chapter: Effective Coaching.

References

Alexander C.M., & Harrison P.J. (2003). Reflex connections from forearm and hand afferents to shoulder girdle muscles in humans. Experimental Brain Research, 148(3), 277-282.

Aman J.E., Elangovan N., Yeh I.-L., & Konczak J. (2015). The effectiveness of proprioceptive training for improving motor function: A systematic review. Frontiers in Human Neuroscience, 8, 1075.

An B., & Woo Y. (2017). Center of mass with the use of smartphone during walking in healthy individuals. Journal of Physical Therapy Science, 29(8), 1426-1428.

Bernardet U., Alaoui S.F., Studd K., Bradley K., Pasquier P., & Schiphorst T. (2019). Assessing the reliability of the Laban Movement Analysis system. PLOS ONE, 14(6), 1-23,

Blozik E., Laptinskaya D., Herrmann-Lingen C., Schaefer H., *et al.* (2009). Depression and anxiety as major determinants of neck pain: A cross-sectional study in general practice. BMC Musculoskeletal Disorders, 10, 13.

Bordoni B., Purgol S., Bizzarri A., Modica M., & Morabito B. (2018). The influence of breathing on the central nervous system. Cureus 10(6), 1-8.

Breedvelt J.J.F., Amanvermez Y., Harrer M., Karyotaki E., Bilbody S., & Bockting C.L.H. (2019). The effects of meditation, yoga, and mindfulness on depression, anxiety, and stress in tertiary education students: A meta-analysis. Frontiers in Psychiatry, 10, 193.

Bruijn S.M., & van Dieen J.H. (2018). Control of human gait stability through foot placement. Journal of the Royal Society Interface, 15(143), 20170816.

Bulbena-Cabre A., & Bulbena A. (2018). Anxiety and joint hypermobility: An unexpected association. Current Psychiatry, 17(4), 15-21.

Chekroud S.R., Gueorguieva R., Zheutlin A.B., Paulus M., *et al.* (2018). Association between physical exercise and mental health in 1·2 million individuals in the USA between 2011 and 2015: A cross-sectional study. Lancet Psychiatry, 5(9), 739-746.

Chevalier G. (2015). The effect of grounding the human body on mood. Psychological Reports, 116(2), 534-542.

Chevalier G., Patel S., Weiss L., Chopra D., & Mills P.J. (2019). The effects of grounding (earthing) on bodyworkers' pain and overall quality of life: A randomized controlled trial. Explore (NY), 15(3), 181-190.

Chevalier G., Sinatra S.T., Oschman J.L., Sokal K., & Sokal P. (2012). Earthing: Health implications of reconnecting the human body to the earth's surface electrons. Journal of Environmental and Public Health, 2012, 291541.

Chow Y.W., & Tsang H.W. (2007). Biopsychosocial effects of qigong as a mindful exercise for people with anxiety disorders: A speculative review. Journal of Alternative Complementary Medicine, 13(8), 831-839.

Cramer H., Lauche R., Anbeter D., Pilkington K., *et al.* (2018). Yoga for anxiety: A systematic review and meta-analysis of randomized controlled trials. Depression and Anxiety, 35(9), 830-843.

De Santis D., Zenzeri J., Casadio M., Masia L., *et al.* (2015). Robot-assisted training of the kinesthetic sense: Enhancing proprioception after stroke. Frontiers in Human Neuroscience, 8, 1037.

Descilo T., Vedamurtachar A., Gerbarg P.L., Nagaraja D., *et al.* (2010). Effects of a yoga breath intervention alone and in combination with an exposure therapy for post-traumatic stress disorder and depression in survivors of the 2004 South-East Asia tsunami. Acta Psychiatrica Scandinavia, 121(4), 289-300.

Doll A., Holzel B.K., Boucard C.C., Wohlschlager A.M., & Sorg C. (2015). Mindfulness is associated with intrinsic functional connectivity between default mode and salience networks. Frontiers in Human Neuroscience, 9, 461.

Eccles J.A., Beacher F.D.C., Gray M.A., & Jones C.L. (2012). Brain structure and joint hypermobility: Relevance to the expression of psychiatric symptoms. British Journal of Psychiatry, 200(6), 508-509.

Fogarty M.J., Mantilla C.B., & Sieck G.C. (2018). Breathing: Motor control of diaphragm muscle. Physiology, 32(2), 113-126.

Geuter U., Heller M.C., & Weaver J.O. (2010). Elsa Gindler and her influence on Wilhelm Reich and body psychotherapy. Body Movement and Dance in Psychotherapy—An International Journal for Theory, Research and Practice, 5(1), 59-73.

Goyal M., Singh S., Sibinga E.M., Gould N.F., *et al.* (2014). Meditation programs for psychological stress and well-being: A systematic review and meta-analysis. JAMA Internal Medicine, 174(3), 357-368.

Gueguen J., Piot M.-A., Orri M., Gutierre A., *et al.* (2017). Group Qigong for adolescent inpatients with anorexia nervosa: Incentives and barriers. PLOS ONE, 12(2), 1-20.

Hagins M., Pietrek M., Sheikhzadeh A., Nordin M., & Axen K. (2004). The effects of breath control on intra-abdominal pressure during lifting tasks. Spine, 29(4), 464-469.

Hansson E.E., Beckman A., & Hakansson A. (2010). Effect of vision, proprioception, and the position of the vestibular organ on postural sway. Acta Oto-Laryngologica, 130(12), 1358-1363.

Hayes J.C., & Kraemer D.J.M. (2017). Grounded understanding of abstract concepts: The case of STEM learning. Cognitive Research: Principles and Implications, 2(71), 7.

Hoffman J., & Gabel C.P. (2015). The origins of Western mind–body exercise methods. Physical Therapy Reviews, 20(5-6), 315-324.

Jolly E., Tamir D.I., Burum B., & Mitchell J.P. (2019). Wanting without enjoying: The social value of sharing experiences. PLOS ONE 14(4), e0215318.

Kennedy P.M., & Inglis J.T. (2002). Distribution and behavior of glamorous cutaneous receptors in the human foot sole. Journal of Physiology, 538(Pt 3), 995-1002.

Konig Ignasiak N., Ravi D.K., Orter S., Hosseini Nasab S.H., Taylor W.R., & Singh N.B. (2019). Does variability of football kinematics correlate with dynamic stability of the centre of mass during walking? PLOS ONE, 14(5), 1-14.

Ku J., Lee Y.S., Kim K.T., Chang H., & Cho Y.W. (2020). Alterations in salience network functional connectivity in individuals with restless leg syndrome. Scientific Reports, 10, 7643.

Lichtenstein M.B., Hinze C.J., Emborg B., Thomsen F., & Hemmingsen S.D. (2017). Compulsive exercise: Links, risks and challenges faced. Psychology Research and Behavior Management, 10, 85-95.

Milanesi R., & Caregnato R.C.A. (2016). Intra-abdominal pressure: An integrative review. Einstein (Sao Paulo), 14(3), 423-430.

Min K.E., Liu P.J., & Kim S. (2017). Sharing extraordinary experiences fosters feelings of closeness. Personality and Social Psychology Bulletin, 44(1), 107-121.

Mitchell K.S., Dick A.M., DiMartino D.M., Smith B.N., et al. (2014). A pilot study of a randomized controlled trial of yoga as an intervention for PTSD symptoms in women. Journal of Trauma and Stress, 27(2), 121-128.

Molnar C., & Gair J. (2015). Concepts of Biology: 1st Canadian Edition. BCcampus. Accessed on December 7, 2022 at https://opentextbc.ca/biology/chapter/20-1-systems-of-gas-exchange.

Mullan K. (2012). The Art and Science of Somatics: Theory, History and Scientific Foundations. MALS Final Projects, 1995–2019. Accessed on January 16, 2023 at https://creativematter.skidmore.edu/mals_stu_schol/89.

Mullan K. (2017). Somatics herstories: Tracing Elsa Gindler's educational antecedents Hade Kallmeyer and Genevieve Stebbins. Journal of Dance and Somatic Practices, 9(2), 159-178.

Neumark-Sztainer D. (2013). Yoga and eating disorders: Is there a place for yoga in the prevention and treatment of eating disorders and disordered eating behaviours? Advances in Eating Disorders Theory, Research, and Practice, 2(2), 136-145.

Nguyen M.H., & Kruse, A. (2012). The effects of Tai Chi training on physical fitness, perceived health, and blood pressure in elderly Vietnamese. Open Access Journal of Sports Medicine, 3, 7-16.

Oliver K.A., & Ashurst J.V. (2018). Anatomy, thorax, phrenic nerves. In: StatPearls [Internet]. Treasure Island, FL: StatPearls Publishing.

Oschman J.L., Chevalier G., & Brown R. (2015). The effects of grounding (earthing) on inflammation, the immune response, wound healing, and prevention and treatment of chronic inflammatory and autoimmune diseases. Journal of Inflammation Research, 8, 83-96.

Peer M., Salomon R., Goldberg I., Blaanke O., & Arzy S. (2015). Brain system for mental orientation in space, time, and person. Proceedings of the National Academy of Sciences of the United States of America, 112(35), 11072-11077.

Proske U., & Gandevia S.C. (2009). The kinesthetic senses. Journal of Physiology, 258(Pt 17), 4139-4146.

Proske U., & Gandevia S.C. (2012). The proprioceptive senses: Their roles in signaling body shape, body position and movement, and muscle force. Physiology Review, 92(4), 1651-1697.

Reid K.F., Bannuru R.R., Wang C., Mori D.L., & Niles B.L. (2019). The effects of tai chi mind-body approach on the mechanisms of gulf war illness: An umbrella review. Integrative Medicine Research, 8(3), 167-172.

Sarlegna F.R., & Sainburg R.L. (2009). The roles of vision and proprioception in the planning of reaching movements. Advances in Experimental Medicine & Biology, 629, 317-335.

Schoeller D., & Dunaetz N. (2018). Thinking emergence as interaffecting: Approaching and contextualizing Eugene Gendlin's Process Method. Continental Philosophy Review, 51, 123-140.

Sharma M., & Haider T. (2015). Tai chi as an alternative and complementary therapy for anxiety: A systematic review. Journal of Evidence-Based Complementary Alternative Medicine, 20(2), 143-153.

Smith A.R., Zuromski K.L., & Dodd D.R. (2018). Eating disorders and suicidality: What we know, what we don't know, and suggestions for future research. Current Opinions in Psychology, 22, 63-67.

Smith T.O., Jerman E., Easton V., Bacon H., et al. (2013). Do people with benign joint hypermobility syndrome (BJHS) have reduced joint proprioception? A systematic review and meta-analysis. Rheumatology International, 33(11), 2709-2716.

Smyth C. (2016). Feldenkrais Method® and health. Feldenkrais Research Journal, 5. Accessed on December 7, 2022 at https://feldenkraisresearchjournal.org/index.php/journal/article/view/23.

Stein B., Stanford T., & Rowland B. (2014). Development of multisensory integration from the perspective of the individual neuron. Nature Reviews Neuroscience 15, 520–535.

Uebelacker L.A., & Broughton M.K. (2016). Yoga for depression and anxiety: A review of published research and implications for healthcare providers. Rhode Island Medical Journal, 99(3), 20-22.

Valenzuela-Moguillansky C., Reyes-Reyes A., & Gaete M.I. (2017). Exteroceptive and interoceptive body-self awareness in fibromyalgia patients. Frontiers in Human Neuroscience, 11, 117.

Wang C., Bannuru R., Ramel J., Kupelnick B., Scott T., & Schmid C.H. (2010). Tai Chi on psychological well-being: A systematic review and meta-analysis. BMC Complementary and Alternative Medicine, 10, 23.

Wang F., Lee E.K., Benson H., Fricchione G., Wang W., & Yeung A.S. (2014). The effects of tai chi on depression, anxiety, and psychological well-being: A systematic review and meta-analysis. International Journal of Behavioral Medicine, 21(4), 605-617.

Watson J. (2013). Knowing through the felt-sense: A gesture of openness to the other. International Journal of Children's Spirituality, 1, 118-130.

Yang G.-Y., Wang L.-Q., Ren J., Zhang Y., et al. (2015). Evidence base of clinical studies on Tai Chi: A bibliometric analysis. PLOS ONE, 10(3), 1-13.

Yin J., & Dishman R.K. (2014). The effect of Tai Chi and Qigong practice on depression and anxiety symptoms: A systematic review and meta-regression analysis of randomized controlled trials. Mental Health and Physical Activity, 7(3), 135-146.

Young C. (2010). The history and development of body-psychotherapy: European diversity. Body Movement and Dance in Psychotherapy, 5(1), 5-19

Zaccaro A., Piarulli A., Laurino M., Garbella M., *et al.* (2018). How breath-control can change your life: A systematic review on psycho-physiological correlates of slow breathing. Frontiers in Human Neuroscience, 12, 353.

Zelano C., Jiang H., Zhou G., Arora N., *et al.* (2016). Nasal respiration entrains human limbic oscillations and modulates cognitive function. Journal of Neuroscience, 36(49), 12448-12467.

Zhang L., Layne C., Lowder T., & Liu J. (2012). A review focused on the psychological effectiveness of Tai Chi on different populations. Evidence-Based Complementary and Alternative Medicine, 2012, 678107.

Zouhal H., Abderrahman A.B., Dupont G., Truptin P., *et al.* (2018). Laterality influences agility performance in elite soccer players. Frontiers in Physiology, 9, 807.

CHAPTER 6

Effective Coaching

A client I hadn't seen in a while contacted me recently for help with her pelvic floor. When she arrived, I asked her how she was doing. She told me things were stressful. The pandemic, work, and the school situation for her children were all adding stress to her life.

I listened, gently suggesting basic floor movements. She continued to talk as she moved. I watched as her nervous system shifted and her posture changed in the way that it does when people start to feel more relaxed.

I moved into more challenging movements as her focus shifted towards her body. She talked little during the middle part of the session; her attention was on moving in interesting ways and feeling connections in various positions.

We finished up with some breath work. "How are you feeling?" I asked.

"So much better than when I came in. My neck pain is gone and my pelvis feels more stable. Thank you."

One of the critical components to improving health of any kind, whether it's mental or physical, is feeling supported. In a coaching/teaching or client/service-provider relationship, if you want the client to feel stronger, more capable, and ultimately more resilient, your role is not only to work with the client to provide an appropriate intervention, but also to act as a supportive partner in the journey.

The role of supportive partner is different than the conventional fitness and movement model of teacher and student, where the teacher is expected to know all of the answers and the student is merely meant to follow along. The word "coach" in a teaching environment was first used as a verb by students in reference to tutors who successfully coached them to their goal of passing exams. (At the time, a coach was a mode of transport, such as a horse-drawn coach, that carried someone to a destination; coaching someone became a metaphor for carrying someone where they wanted to go (Dictionary.com, 2022).)

The word "teach" comes from the old English word "tæcan," which means to show, present, persuade, or declare (Online Etymology Dictionary, 2022). "Laeran," which is the source for the modern words "learn" and "lore," meant to teach, guide, or instruct. If our clients come to us with specific goals related to movement, whether it's to establish a mind/body connection, get stronger, or learn a specific skill, our role is to facilitate an environment where they have an opportunity to learn. This becomes less about our ability to persuade, declare, or demonstrate our expertise and more about the client's experience. The first step towards making the experience more about the client and less about our beliefs and agendas is cultivating active listening.

Listening, like all forms of interpersonal communication, is a skill that can be developed through reflection and attention. We talked about active listening in Chapter 4, but let's review and explore the concept more fully.

Active listening is considered a therapeutic micro-skill that makes a client feel heard through attentively listening and empathically responding. Researchers agree that it has four main components: expressing interest in the speaker's message through non-verbal involvement, paraphrasing the speaker's message, refraining from judgment, and encouraging the speaker to elaborate on their beliefs or feelings by asking questions. It has been proposed that active listening demonstrates empathy and builds trust (Weger *et al.*, 2014).

Research suggests that active listening is beneficial in a variety of settings, including in medical professions, education, and therapeutic settings (Jahromi *et al.*, 2016; Weger *et al.*, 2014). In a patient-centered care model, healthcare that focuses on the patient's needs and desires and emphasizes listening to the patient so that they feel heard, respected, and understood leads to better patient outcomes. Active listening may also contribute to better self-management of blood pressure and weight control (Haley *et al.*, 2017). In a study of nursing students, active listening and self-awareness were significantly associated with empathy (*ibid.*). Both active listening and self-awareness are skills that can be improved, and may have a positive impact on patient outcomes because they place the emphasis on the patient, not the medical professional.

American psychologist Carl Rogers, whose work was the first to include a patient-centered or client-centered approach to therapy, defined empathy as the ability to understand, recognize, and share a person's experience (Rogers, 1957). Self-awareness is a trait that is related to the understanding of the self and the impact that decisions and behavior have on both the self and others. Individuals who perform self-reflective reasoning tend to have higher levels of self-awareness. Developing empathy and self-awareness can be done through practice and self-reflection (Dishon *et al.*, 2017). When I was with the client I mentioned at the beginning of the chapter, I listened as she spoke and reflected some of the story back to her in a conversational way. I made it very clear from the beginning of our time together that the session was about her and what she needed. Sometimes, feeling better is about moving differently or more; sometimes, it's about feeling heard.

When you reflect upon the complexity of sensations like pain, the importance of being heard and the impact that has on a person's sense of emotional and physical health and well-being shouldn't be surprising. Researchers suggest that empathy evolved to allow us to form and maintain social bonds; these bonds are necessary for survival and maintaining a general sense of well-being. Empathy affects several areas of the brain, including the amygdala, which, as we saw in Chapter 1, is involved in our perception of safety. It also impacts the central executive network, or conscious awareness, and the parts of the brain associated with caregiving, such as the brainstem and the hypothalamus (Decety & Fotopoulou, 2014).

If the first step to effective coaching is creating an environment where the client feels heard and the provider (teacher, coach, clinician) is demonstrating empathy through self-awareness and active listening, how can these skills be integrated?

Let's return to the original idea of active listening and further break down what it is and isn't. Before we move on, take a moment to write down: a) whether you think you are currently a good listener and b) why you are (or aren't) a good listener.

In a large review published in *Harvard Business Review* (Zenger & Folkman, 2016), the authors summarized that most people think good listening is based on three basic things:

- Not talking when someone is speaking.
- Using facial expressions and the appropriate verbal responses to let the person talking know you are listening.
- Being able to repeat, almost verbatim, what the person talking has said.

However, when the data of 3942 participants in a development program to help managers become better coaches was analyzed, the most effective listeners didn't necessarily simply reflect back what had just been said or not interrupt while someone else was speaking. The best listeners periodically asked questions that promoted insight and self-discovery, making the conversation a two-person experience. The best listeners made the conversation positive for the other person, creating a safe environment that made them feel supported. Good listening wasn't about using silence to prepare a response or point out flaws in a person's logic; rather, good listeners facilitated conversations that flowed smoothly, in a non-defensive way. Finally, good listeners made suggestions, providing feedback in a positive way that opened up alternative paths or ideas to consider. (The researchers point out that one of the requirements for feedback to be taken in a non-critical way may be that the person demonstrates good listening skills throughout the conversation, making suggestions more credible and have less of a judgmental feeling (Zenger & Folkman, 2016).

Focused Attention

Active listening requires paying attention. If you are focused on something else, whether it's teaching something a specific way, what you are going to say next, or what you are having for lunch later, you will not be focusing your attention on the person in front of you. One aspect of listening is non-verbal communication. Non-verbal communication is what you say during the space between words and includes facial expression and body movement. It accounts for approximately 80 percent of the essential communication between individuals, and researchers split it into four distinct categories:

- Kinesics, which refers to head and body movements.

- Vocalics, which is non-linguistic vocal cues, like pitch and volume.
- Haptics, aka body contact.
- Proxemics, which are body cues. How far away do you stand from the client? How do you orient your body while talking to the client? (Liu *et al.*, 2016)

(I wrote this before the Covid pandemic. It will be interesting to see if the way we communicate non-verbally changes in the upcoming years. Standing less than six feet away from a client, for instance, might be a thing of the past. But how does that change how we interpret and relate to each other? I don't know the answer, but it's interesting to consider.)

If you simply watch someone as they interact with you, you can pick up several non-verbal cues. Observing the positions they find most efficient or comfortable can tell you something about their movement habits, their comfort level with you, how interested they are in what they are doing, whether their body is craving something else, or if they are experiencing any physical discomfort. Attention to these sorts of nuances requires focus; if you aren't used to focusing for long periods of time or you know you don't have the ability to focus for more than a specific amount of time, it's important to take this information into account when you are scheduling clients. If you are providing a service that requires you to pay attention and actively listen, it is unfair on the client if they come in when you aren't able to focus and provide the level of attention that supports their experience (just ask my clients who come in at 4:00 p.m. on a Friday—my focus is less sharp than it is at 10:30 a.m. on a Monday).

You can develop focused attention through activities that require sustained focus. Meditations that focus on breathing are an easy way to begin building attention. Game play or externally based tasks can develop focused attention (examples will be discussed further in Chapter 9). Learning and educating both require paying attention for a longer duration. Whether it's learning a musical instrument, teaching someone a foreign language, or deciphering research on listening so that it can be applied in a practical way, the ability to accomplish the task requires focus. Developing your listening skills begins with developing your ability to pay attention.

Judging

Active listening is not judging. Judging is characterized by the natural tendency to evaluate from a personal frame of reference and may include behaviors like criticizing, name calling, or diagnosing (Robertson, 2005).

This, of course, is challenging when people ask specific questions about why things are the way they are and you want to provide an answer. It's human nature to want to help or fix in order to make someone feel better. Unfortunately, this type of behavior isn't conducive to an active listening environment and may affect your client's perception of whether you are able to feel empathetic towards their situation. In fact, always telling creates more of a power differential, where the client no longer views the clinician as a supportive partner in their quest towards improved well-being but instead as an expert who knows all of the answers. This doesn't instill a sense of autonomy or confidence, both of which are beneficial for improving strength and well-being.

Other potential roadblocks to active listening include offering advice, asking excessive questions, or reassuring. While well intentioned, these types of communication don't give the client an opportunity to work out the solution on their own.

Pretend you are working with someone who is scared to squat because they have heard it's bad for their knees. Since they have knee pain occasionally, they don't want to make it worse with exercise.

Being the well-educated movement professional that you are, you realize that squatting is a function of daily life and research does not support the idea that squatting is injurious to the knees (Cotter *et al.*, 2014). You promptly cite research in order to debunk this myth and have the client come into a squat position, using five different instructions in order to help the client distribute force throughout the lower extremity so you can further prove that squatting isn't going to do any damage to the knees. After performing six repetitions, you have the client rest. How do you think the client feels?

Probably not very good—on several levels. Instead of having an experience of building trust and rapport through two-way communication, active listening, and empathy, the client had their concerns ignored because, in this hypothetical situation, you, the movement professional, judged the situation and the client's concerns, "fixing" the problem through science and movement.

What if instead of having them squat, you listen to the client and ask if it would be okay to work on different ways to get up out of a chair? If the client says that would be fine, instead of having them stand up right away, what if you ask them to press the feet strongly into the ground until they feel work in the upper legs? Do you think the client's experience would be different?

Yes—this scenario builds trust, increases neuroception because you aren't asking the client to do something they deem potentially harmful, and gives you an opportunity to help the client feel different parts of themselves. This will improve their confidence in their physical body, increase proprioception, and with time, reduce fear of trying different movements.

We will discuss ideas for regressions and improving a sense of safety in positions in Chapter 7, but for now, consider that if your idea of what your client needs is directly opposed to your client's beliefs and the client is fearful of or anxious about movement in any way, pushing your own agenda on to your client is not acting from a place of service. Remember earlier in the chapter when I mentioned that active listening in a medical setting was associated with a decrease in blood pressure and weight? This implies that the subjects who were the recipients of active listening were more willing to make long-term behavior changes that, ultimately, led to an improvement in health outcomes that would impact their lives. If the goal is to impact a person's overall well-being, taking the time to improve listening skills is an important part of helping the client feel supported.

We are all human. It's difficult to be an empathetic listener 100 percent of the time. I know on days when I have worked with eight different clients and my sister or my husband want to have a conversation with me, I have a difficult time focusing and being as engaged with them as I would like to be. (Because I am generally a good listener, they can both tell when my listening skills are subpar and call me out on it.) Taking the time to develop your listening skills will improve rapport with clients and improve the client's confidence in both you and their physical abilities.

Self-Awareness and Presence

Presence can refer to a number of things. There is spatial presence, which is where you are physically located in space in relation to other people. Social presence is the feeling of being with other people and the sense of social interaction. Co-presence is the feeling of being together with others, even though people are in separate places (think virtual reality or computer-generated experiences) (Ling *et al.*, 2014).

In a movement setting, presence functions spatially—where you and your client are in relation to each other—and socially—does the client feel like they are actually with you, or have either of you mentally checked out so you're there but not really there?

Social presence is determined by two components: intimacy and immediacy. Intimacy refers to how connected two people feel during a conversation and immediacy is the psychological distance between the two people communicating (Oh *et al.*, 2018). Intimacy and immediacy are both conveyed through non-verbal cues, such as touch, face, body, and voice. Non-verbal social cues are largely involuntary and allow the recipient to accurately gauge the person's emotions and/or attitudes (Gilboa-Schechtman & Shachar-Lavie, 2013).

For the professional, this means paying attention to how the client is responding non-verbally to what you are saying. What they are doing can provide insight into whether the movement intervention is the right choice for that person on that day. Modifying or altering a movement intervention based on a person's response is a way to increase the likelihood of a positive outcome. This is different from a client walking in and saying they do not feel like doing anything physical, only to announce 45 minutes later, "I feel *so* much better. I am really glad I came." I am referring to the words or exercises that may elicit feelings of frustration, irritation, or annoyance. When those show up, it's important that the movement professional has the ability to reroute and find something the client can mentally engage with in a more positive way.

Individuals with PTSD may dissociate, which means they may feel either separate from their own body or like they are in a place that is strange and unfamiliar (Boyd *et al.*, 2018). Dissociation causes a sense of disconnectedness from the environment, the body, and the other person in the room. A person who is dissociated isn't present, and the lack of presence can be felt by both individuals.

While dissociation may have originally been a coping mechanism, it often accompanies altered fear learning in individuals with PTSD (Seligowski *et al.*, 2019).

Pretend you are balancing on rails that are four feet off the ground with a group of people. Though you practiced on 2x4s (pieces of plywood) earlier in the day, the rails are narrower and in a position that could be dangerous if you lose your footing. You experience an increase in heart rate and feel uncertain about transferring from a crouched position to a full stand. You go slowly, assessing the safety of the situation before determining whether you feel comfortable standing all of the way up.

In contrast, Nick, one of the members of the group, stands up on the rail, skipping the crouching position altogether. He doesn't look fully in control, and there is a blank look on his face, as though he isn't completely present or aware of what he is doing. He begins walking unsteadily, his breathing slows, and there is no sign of fear on his face. One plausible explanation is that he is dissociating, which is suppressing his fear response, even though the situation would be considered scary or higher risk by most (unless, of course, you have been practicing walking on progressively higher rails throughout the day—then the assessment of risk would be low because it would be a familiar situation; for the purposes of this example, let's say Nick has no previous experience of walking on rails until this exact moment).

While Nick was likely dissociating, the reverse can also happen. Someone can become hyperaroused, fully activating the SNS, and unable to recalibrate and find the optimal amount of arousal needed for the task at hand. Your ability to stay in tune with your client's experience, notice their reactions, and listen to their words and actions will help you know when a task is appropriately challenging or when you need to switch gears and give their nervous system a chance to regulate.

I have witnessed the sudden disappearance of clients as they retreat to their default mode networks and lose their hold on the present moment. It happens to everyone once in a while and can be exacerbated by stress, lack of sleep, or general anxiety. Anchoring the client in the present moment through a kinesthetic focal point, like asking them to feel the ground or giving them an externally based task like reaching for a specific object that's in an awkward position, can bring them back, re-establishing their spatial and social presence.

For the practitioner, maintaining presence is a practice, requiring self-reflection and self-awareness. It is easy to get caught up in the next instruction or what you want the client to do next; it's also easy to get so caught up in the client's physical expression of a specific exercise that you forget to check in with their overall experience. If your goal is to make something look a certain way or to find a specific position, the client as a person can get lost. Finding a balance between physical instructions and giving the client space to explore is part of the learning process. If your goal is to create client empowerment and autonomy, saying less will actually create more impact (we'll discuss this in further detail later in this chapter). Before we move on, think about the last session you had with a client. How much time did you spend instructing? How much time did you spend listening and observing the client's non-verbal cues?

Self-Reflection

The questions above are a way to self-reflect. Self-reflection is an important process that assists with learning. It enables you to critically appraise what happened in the past in a specific circumstance. This gives you an opportunity to identify what you could potentially change to create a different outcome (Helyer, 2015).

Self-reflection is different than self-criticism. When you reflect, you aren't using negative self-talk or over-emphasizing perceived flaws. You are simply observing, without judgment, your performance. I self-reflect after every workshop and every session, assessing what I could have done better and what went well. Sitting down and thinking about whether changing your behavior, words, or how you instruct serves to make you better. You learn to recognize your mistakes and identify things you could do differently. As a result, you try things differently next time, until you begin to hone in on what teaching style leads to the best outcomes.[1]

Self-reflection, also referred to as critical reflection in some of the literature, is considered a metacognitive skill. This means you consciously try to control the cognitive process before, during, or after events where you are learning or communicating (Patterson, 2011). It's considered a key component of critical thinking and is part of both experiential and transformative learning processes (Kim *et al.*, 2018).

---

[1] There is, of course, an individualized component to this since not everyone will resonate with the same words and teaching style. But reflecting on what worked and what didn't coupled with the willingness to try new ways of teaching will make you more adaptable and better able to recognize the teaching style that best works for the person (or people) you are with.

Learning to self-reflect also makes it easier to help your clients self-reflect. When you understand the process and how to direct attention after an experience, your clients will become more engaged and present, learning rather than simply going through the movements.

EXERCISE: SELF-REFLECTION IN MOVEMENT

Come into a quadruped position. Rock your torso forward and back eight times.

When you finish, come into a comfortable seated position. How did you rock forward and back? Did you use your hands or your knees to direct the movement? Or did you move just your torso without paying attention to your hands and knees?

If you aren't sure, rock back and forth on your hands and knees a few more times, paying attention to what allows you to move your torso back and forth.

When you have a clear idea of what you use to move your torso, pause in a comfortable seated position. What position was your head in while you were rocking forward and back? Was it hanging down? Extended so your eyes could look out? Or was it somewhere in between?

If you aren't sure, perform a few more, observing the position of your head. Once you have a clear idea of your head, pause in a comfortable seated position.

Finally, do you round or arch your spine while you rock back, or do you keep your spine position fairly unchanged? Another way to say this is do you move at your hips, or does your spine move to allow you to rock back?

If you aren't sure, perform a few more. Once you have a clear idea of how you perform the movement, rest.

How did that go? Did you learn anything about how you perform the movement of rocking forward and back when you aren't thinking about it? Did you get any ideas for how you could try rocking forward and back differently? Can you see how this is different than talking as the movement is happening?

This isn't to say that instructing as the movement is happening is wrong; it isn't. Augmented feedback (which is the type of feedback that is given by an outside source, such as a coach or teacher) has a time and a place and is an aspect of skill learning (Schmidt, 1991). However, teaching people how to reflect and that it is okay to reflect will increase their overall awareness outside of their time with you. It reminds them that their situation isn't permanent and that they have choice in how they move and how they experience situations. As you will see later in this chapter, when you are working with individuals who experience fear around movement or chronic-pain types of situations, this can be valuable.

This also can also help spark curiosity and interest in movement. "What happens if I try this a different way?" is one of the most valuable questions a person can ask themselves when they are dealing with a painful situation that feels permanent.

A (Brief) Review of Motor Learning

When you are teaching someone a new skill, the very first time they see or hear the skill being explained will require focus. As they perform the skill, it will probably feel awkward, and initially it won't be efficient. This is the cognitive stage of motor learning and is characterized by high variability of performance and errors. During this stage, feedback is integrated continuously and extra instruction may be required to direct the learner towards ways to make the movement feel more smooth and coordinated (Politis, 2018).

After a bit of practice, the skill will become more fluid. There will be fewer errors and there will be less obvious variability of the skill. The mechanisms of the skill become more consolidated, and the learner becomes more confident in their ability to perform the skill consistently. Less feedback and instruction is required. This is the associative stage.

At some point, the learner no longer has to think consciously about performing the skill. It begins to occur automatically in a consistent and less variable way. It's efficient and can be performed while doing other things. This is the autonomous stage.

Different parts of the brain are activated during different stages of learning. During the cognitive stage, the high amount of concentration and focus required activates the frontal and parietal areas; when learning becomes consolidated, long-lasting neuronal changes likely occur. This should make sense when you think back to what you learned in

Chapter 2—when neurons consistently fire together, over time, a neural network is created and the strength of the connection between the neurons becomes stronger. This formation of a memory about how to perform an activity takes place both during and after practice; in fact, sleep is believed to be a key factor in the brain's ability to consolidate memories (Brem, Ran, & Pascual-Leone, 2013). Your client's ability to progress may actually be helped or hindered by whether they consistently access rapid eye movement (REM) sleep.

Because learning is dependent on a variety of factors, how you impart the information will play a role in your client's sense of success, whether the experience is rewarding, and your client's mindset around the activity.

The Interpretation of Language

How you deliver instructions can alter a client's perception of how to perform a specific skill. The language you use can induce confidence or spark fear. It can make a skill feel easy or challenging, and it can make the client feel empowered or unable. Considering the words you choose when you deliver instruction can influence a client's mental and physical experience.

"Embodied cognition" is a broad term that describes how we acquire and represent knowledge through the mind and the body. When we process language, we use sensorimotor information attained through experience to understand the concepts behind the words. It has been suggested by some researchers that embodiment exists on a spectrum and is, perhaps, more important for processing certain concepts than others (Wellsby & Pexman, 2014).

For instance, how much embodiment is necessary to comprehend abstract ideas such as differential equations? These ideas are largely cognitive, requiring no body awareness or motor comprehension, so probably not very much.

How much embodiment is required to understand ideas that affect our relationship with the immediate environment, such as how to put a baby's car seat in the car, how to cook dinner for four people, or how to interact with someone who has a terminal illness? All of these skills require an essence of embodiment, and when we learn about these skills, whether they are from a how-to manual, a podcast, or a lecture on the topic, we experience the words with more than just cognitive thought. The instructional words are felt with the entire body and, arguably, the more embodied you are, the more you experience the words in a multisensory way.

The idea that language processing and cognition is influenced by a number of senses is supported by the fact that gesturing has been shown to facilitate language processing. When we watch someone else perform an action, mirror neurons fire, creating a connection between us and the person performing the movement. We are also more likely to remember specific cognitive tasks when we use our bodies in the learning process (Wilson & Foglia, 2017). Using words that appeal to a client's senses, then, may improve understanding and enhance neuroception, enabling the client to more accurately perform the task in a focused way.

Metaphors that relate to something the client has previous experience with and spatial instructions that clearly place the body in relation to the environment are both examples of using language as tools to enhance understanding. Choosing relevant examples and using specific directional instructions make a new task feel less daunting and more familiar. This becomes particularly important when you are teaching a skill to someone that they initially find unattainable or intimidating because there is fear involved, or when you are asking someone to perform a skill that is foreign to them and completely unfamiliar in their body. The words you use to convey instructions are intimately related to a client's success and sense of autonomy.

A (Very Short) Overview of the Psychology of Behavior

It has been suggested that there are three main theories that govern behavior change: self-efficacy theory, self-determination theory, and self-regulation theory (Garrin, 2014).

We saw in Chapter 2 that self-efficacy is the ability to take steps to achieve targeted goals, which is determined by the belief that changing a behavior will change an outcome.

Self-determination is a self-sustaining form of motivation that is guided by inner drive. Self-determined individuals internalize a desire for competence, believe they are in charge of their destinies (so they believe they are autonomous), and tend to assimilate or relate to others, which means social support is an aspect to self-determination.

Self-regulation is the ability to moderate thoughts and emotions. The ability to self-regulate has direct links to motivation; social support appears to be predictive of the self-regulatory behaviors necessary for exercise adherence.

Your words and client interactions can increase an individual's sense of autonomy, competency, and mastery. They can be supportive and improve adherence in positive behaviors associated with exercise and movement. They can help people create long-term changes that will benefit their emotional and physical well-being.

"Fine," you may be thinking. "My words matter, but you've been talking about this for a while with no concrete examples." Let's look at how these ideas play out in a movement setting.

Inspiring Autonomy and Mastery

Do you give your clients the tools to feel autonomous and feel like they have mastery over their physical abilities?

Creating mastery and autonomy in a movement setting is done by showing and giving options. Let's look at this.

Pretend you are working with a woman who has chronic low back pain. She was referred to you by a medical professional, her MRI shows no structural issues in her back, and she is both skeptical and tired. She has tried other forms of exercise and movement therapy, including Pilates, physical therapy, and yoga, and she equates exercise with more pain.

You ask her to stand up from a chair without using her hands, and she tells you it hurts her back. What do you do?

We have explored this action of standing up from a chair repeatedly in the preceding chapters, so you may already have some ideas about how to explore this specific action.

You could abort the exercise and say something along the lines of "If it hurts, you should avoid doing it." The problem with this is it feeds into the idea that if something is painful, it may cause more tissue damage and should be avoided at all costs, which isn't necessarily true. It can also cause some clients to adopt an avoidant strategy towards movement—if they think a movement will cause pain, they avoid it at all possible costs.

There are, of course, situations where movements should be avoided. I remove things occasionally when it is apparent the progression was too quick and the client needs to spend more time working on the fundamental components of the skill. However, I return to the progression eventually, when the client is more prepared, teaching the client (hopefully) that the goal isn't avoidance; rather, it's adequate preparation.

With a low-load activity like getting out of a chair without using the hands, there are positional instructions that can be used to alter the client's experience of the exercise. Asking this client to push her feet into the floor without standing up, for instance, could help her feel the support of the ground beneath her. You could also ask the client to imagine that there is a string lightly pulling the anterior superior iliac spine (ASIS—the two front hip bones) together as she exhales and presses the feet into the floor. This instruction will give her a sense of center; usually between the grounding and the centering, the feeling in the low back disappears.

Or you could place a soft medium-sized ball between the client's knees for her to hold lightly and give her a light to medium-weight to hold as she stands up. This would change her relationship to the task; another way to do this would be to ask her to toss a tennis ball in the air and catch it standing up. As the goals change (don't drop the ball between the knees and hold the light weight, or catch a ball as I stand up), so does the person's strategy around how they perform the movement.

You could also have the client pull herself up using her hands on stall bars or with rings or a stable strap. This can build confidence in the action of transferring weight from sitting to standing in a way that is different from using the hands to push down into a chair to come up.

It's also important for you, the practitioner, to remember that noise occurs in the PNS during all stages of learning, but especially during the cognitive stage.

Remember how neurons are given either an electrical or chemical signal to fire? Sometimes, even though they are given the signal to fire, they don't, or more neurons fire than is necessary. This noise is what causes variation within movement (Hasson *et al.*, 2016). It's the reason that even though you have walked up the steps to your front door thousands of times, one Tuesday morning, you accidentally misstep and catch your foot. Or, when you reach for a glass, an activity you have done countless times throughout your life, you feel a weird zing through your elbow; when you reach for the glass a moment later, the zing is gone (Lee *et al.*, 2016). Noise is normal, and while it is minimized with practice, it still exists.

When someone is first learning how to do something, there is a lot of noise. As a skill becomes more autonomous, the noise significantly lessens and the ability to perform the skill becomes more predictable. When we asked the client to stand up from the chair without using her hands, we could assume she stands up from chairs regularly without thinking about it. You interrupted an unconscious activity and asked her to change how she usually stands up from the chair. This is, understandably, confusing for the nervous system; performing an automatic activity consciously requires more thinking power in order to do something that is generally easy. Changing the focus to something like the feet creates a greater sense of connection between something supporting the body (in this case, the floor) and the body's response to that support.

When you demonstrate to a client that pain during a low-level skill can be altered when they change position or do it a different way, you are giving them an opportunity to feel stronger and more capable. The client begins to understand that experiencing pain with movement can be temporary and that they have more control than they realized over how they move. This instills a greater sense of control and autonomy over the physical body, uniting the client's consciousness with their physicality.

The words you choose are an important part of the process. I like to phrase my words as an inquiry, inviting curiosity to see what happens. I can't know for sure what will happen, since I am not in the client's body, and asking rather than telling invites reflection. "What happens if you press your feet strongly into the ground, like you are pushing the floor away from you to stand up, but you don't actually stand up? What do you experience?"

If I ask this question and the client says they feel work in the legs and nothing in the low back, I might become enthusiastic and then add, "Now try placing your fingers on your two front hip bones. Imagine that there is a line gently tightening, pulling the two front hip bones towards each other. How does that feel?" If the client says they feel their abdominals, I might get even more enthusiastic and start jumping and clapping, because I get really excited about these subtle shifts.

As we have seen, there are different ways to alter a person's experience of standing up. Addressing rib position by using a verbal instruction or by asking the person to hold a weighted object connects the client to center. Drawing attention to the feet can help the person feel more grounded. Using the breath and exhaling (or inhaling) in a specific way to stand up reminds the person to breathe and can also be centering (and activate a different stabilizing system). Using the arms to pull up and out of the chair is a safe way to explore weight transfer and instill confidence.

What matters is that the person begins to realize that they have options and they don't have to experience the movement of standing up just one way. When you phrase the options as inquiries, opportunities to explore "what might happen if...," it gives the client an opportunity to become curious as they realize that their way of moving isn't fixed. It's a fluid state, full of opportunities.

When someone is first learning a new motor skill, or they are learning a new approach to an old motor skill, a number of cognitive processes take place (hence the early stages of motor learning are called the cognitive phases). Learning requires memorization of an internal representation of the movement, that is, what does the movement look like? This allows the sensorimotor system to build a motor program. A motor program is what needs to happen to execute the skill. It also shifts the input that the nervous system is paying attention to so it can generate defined sensory references of the movement before it's executed (Muratori *et al.*, 2013).

Success and replication of a motor pattern occur through the processing of sensory feedback from the nervous system via movement-related information. The outcome of the movement that was performed is compared with the movement goal. This is called "knowledge of results" and leads to improvement of movement control through improving efficiency of the sensorimotor loops (Sharma *et al.*, 2016).

When I was learning how to do tricep dips on the rings, I couldn't figure out how to lower myself down without using my feet to press back up. One day, after weeks of trying to understand how to execute the movement, the ring straps were strung tautly between my feet and the floor. This was purely accidental, and I was far too lazy to fix them, so I left them, assuming I would maneuver my feet around them.

As soon as my feet hit the straps, I felt my upper body responding by pushing. This sent me back up to the starting position. I tried this a few more times (and over a few more days). When I removed the feedback of the strap, I was pleasantly surprised that I suddenly "knew" how to push myself back up without my feet touching the ground. Without the straps, I didn't have enough information about how to coordinate when to push back up. The sensory feedback of the straps gave my brain information it didn't have before, and because I was successful, I was able to replicate the situation.

I figured this all out without any verbal feedback from a coach. Would verbal feedback have helped? Maybe, but it would depend on when and how feedback was given. When you are first learning how to do a movement, there is a lot of processing going on. If someone is talking to you while you are trying to figure things out, you suddenly have to process the words and figure out how to apply the words to the movement you are doing. This means that while verbal feedback is an effective way to focus attention and smooth out movement patterns, it can also interfere with cognitive processes if too much information is given or the instructions aren't clear. The coach's role is to be clear and not overwhelm the client with excessive words while they are trying to learn new movement skills.

It turns out that when it comes to motor learning and verbal instruction, research indicates that verbal instruction should be kept short and simple. For individuals learning a new motor skill, the words chosen should be information dense but still concise. Verbal instruction that accompanies a visual demonstration appears to be effective for retention of complex skills, possibly because when we have a mental image of a physical task, the words carry more meaning than if they were used by themselves (Williams and Hodges, 2004). This means that if you are asking a client to do a shrimp squat, demonstrating it while pointing out the areas you want them to focus on might be more effective than having them do a shrimp squat and instructing them while they are doing the movement.

Embracing fewer words when you teach not only leads to a higher chance the client will retain the skill, it also gives the client an opportunity to figure things out on their own. When things are veering off course, a verbal instruction that focuses attention or uses a metaphorical image the client can relate to re-establishes a connection with what the skill should feel/look like.

EXERCISE: WORD MINIMALISM

Pick a movement task you teach regularly. Write down the exercise exactly as you normally teach it. How many steps are there in your explanation?

If you had to reduce the number of steps by two, how would you alter your explanation? What would you change?

Using fewer words creates less distraction and, for anxious clients, can remove the sense that there is a "right" or "wrong" way to do the exercise, because it gives them space to self-organize. Learning to regain trust in the body's ability to move without being reliant on being told how to move rebuilds confidence and translates into changes in movements outside the studio or gym, which we will explore in Chapter 9.

EXERCISE: SELF-REFLECTION

Film yourself working with a client. Observe how the client responds to you. Are you present and focused on the client?

When you play back the session, listen to your instructions and perform the movement skills, following along with your recorded session. Are your instructions clear? How do the words or directions you use feel in your body? How does your client respond to your words? Is there anything you could change?

This drill can be uncomfortable, especially if you don't like the sound of your voice, the way you look on camera, or self-reflection in general. However, it is important to remember that observation without judgment is a skill, just like focused attention is a skill. The ability to reflect, observe, and fairly assess what you could improve upon (and we all have something to improve upon) is valuable. Additionally, if you want to teach your clients how to self-reflect, it's important that you have practiced self-reflection—that you've tried it on and felt its uncomfortableness, and the challenge of it, and, ultimately, experienced its benefits.

References

Boyd J.E., Protopopescu A., O'Connor C., Neufeld R.W.J., *et al.* (2018). Dissociative symptoms mediate the relation between PTSD symptoms and functional impairment in a sample of military members, veterans, and first responders with PTSD. European Journal of Psychotraumatology, 9(1), 1463794.

Brem A-K., Ran K., & Pascual-Leone A. (2013). Chapter 55: Learning and memory, 693-737. In: Lozano A.M., & Hallett M. (eds) Brain Stimulation Handbook of Clinical Neurology, Vol. 116 (3rd Series).

Cotter J.A., Chaudhari A.M., Jamison S.T., & Devor S.T. (2014). Knee joint kinetics in relation to commonly prescribed squat loads and depths. Journal of Strength & Conditioning Research, 27(7), 1765-1774.

Decety J., & Fotopoulou A. (2014). Why empathy has a beneficial impact on others in medicine: Unifying theories. Frontiers in Behavioral Neuroscience, 8, 457.

Dictionary.com (2022). Coach. Accessed on December 7, 2022 at www.dictionary.com/browse/coach.

Dishon N., Oldmeadow J.A., Critchley C., & Kaufman J. (2017). The effect of trait self-awareness, self-reflection, and perceptions of choice meaningfulness on indicators of social identity within a decision-making context. Frontiers in Psychology, 8, 2934.

Garrin J.M. (2014). Self-efficacy, self-determination, and self-regulation: The role of the fitness professional in social change. Journal of Social Change, 6(1), 41-54.

Gilboa-Schechtman E., & Shachar-Lavie I. (2013). More than a face: A unified theoretical perspective on nonverbal social cue processing in social anxiety. Frontiers in Human Neuroscience, 7, 904.

Haley B., Heo S., Wright P., Barone C., Rettiganti M.R., & Anders M. (2017). Relationships among active listening, self-awareness, empathy, and patient-centered care in associate and baccalaureate degree nursing students. NursingPlus Open 3, 11-16.

Hasson C.J., Gelina O., & Woo G. (2016). Neural control adaptation to motor noise manipulation. Frontiers in Human Neuroscience, 10, 59.

Helyer, R. (2015). Learning through reflection: The critical role of reflection in work-based learning (WBL). Journal of Work-Applied Management, 7(1), 15-27.

Jahromi V.K., Tabatabaee S.S., Abdar Z.E., & Rajabi M. (2016). Active listening: The key of successful communication in hospital managers. Electronic Physician, 8(3), 2123-2128.

Kim Y.H., Kim S.H., & Shin S. (2018). Effects of a work-based critical reflection program for novice nurses. BMC Medical Education, 18(1), 30.

Lee L., Joshua M., Medina J.F., & Lisberger S.G. (2016). Signal, noise, and variation in neural and sensory-motor latency. Neuron, 90(1), 165-176.

Ling Y., Nefs H.T., Morina N., Heynderickx I., & Brinkman W.-P. (2014). A meta-analysis on the relationship between self-reported presence and anxiety in virtual reality exposure therapy for anxiety disorders. PLOS ONE, 9(5), 1-12.

Liu C., Calvo R.A., & Lim R. (2016). Improving medical students' awareness of their non-verbal communication through automated non-verbal behavior feedback. Frontiers in ICT, 3, 11.

Muratori L.M., Lamberg E.M., Quinn L., & Duff S.V. (2013). Applying principles of motor learning and control to upper extremity rehabilitation. Journal of Hand Therapy, 26(2), 94-103.

Oh C.S., Bailenson J.N., & Welch G.F. (2018). A systematic review of social presence: Definition, antecedents, and implications. Frontiers in Robotics and AI, 5, 114.

Online Etymology Dictionary (2022). Teach. Accessed on December 7, 2022 at www.etymonline.com/search?q=teach.

Patterson J. (2011). Metacognitive Skills, 1583-1584. In: Kreutzer J.S., DeLuca J., Caplan B. (eds) Encyclopedia of Clinical Neuropsychology. New York, NY: Springer.

Politis M. (2018). Imaging in Movement Disorders: Imaging Methodology and Applications in Parkinson's Disease. Cambridge, MA: Elsevier.

Robertson K. (2005). Active listening: More than just paying attention. Australian Family Physician, 34(12), 1053-1055.

Rogers C.R. (1957). The necessary and sufficient conditions of therapeutic personality change. Journal of Consulting Psychology, 21(2), 95–103.

Schmidt R.A. (1991). Frequent Augmented Feedback Can Degrade Learning: Evidence and Interpretations, 59-75. In: Requin J., & Stelmach G.E. (eds) Tutorials in Motor Neuroscience. NATO ASI Series (Series D: Behavioural and Social Sciences), Volume 62. Dordrecht: Springer.

Seligowski A.V., Lebois L.A.M., Hill S.B., Kahhale I., et al. (2019). Autonomic responses to fear conditioning among women with PTSD and dissociation. Depression and Anxiety, 36(7), 625-634.

Sharma D.A., Chevidikunnan M.F., Khan F.R., & Gaowgzeh R.A. (2016). Effectiveness of knowledge of result and knowledge of performance in learning of a skilled motor activity by healthy young adults. Journal of Physical Therapy Science, 28(5), 1482-1486.

Weger Jr. H., Bell G.C., Minei E.M., & Robinson M.C. (2014). The relative effectiveness of active listening in initial interactions. International Journal of Listening, 28(1), 13-31.

Wellsby M., & Pexman P.M. (2014). Developing embodied cognition: Insights from children's concepts and language procession. Frontiers in Psychology, 5, 506.

Williams A.M., & Hodges N.J. (2004). Chapter 8: Instructions, Demonstrations, and the Learning Process. Creating and Constraining Options, 145-175. In: Skill Acquisition in Sport: Research, Theory and Practice. Abingdon: Routledge Publishers.

Wilson, R.A. and Foglia, L. (2017). Embodied Cognition. In: Zalta E.N. (ed.) The Stanford Encyclopedia of Philosophy. Accessed on December 7, 2022 at https://plato.stanford.edu/archives/spr2017/entries/embodied-cognition.

Zenger J., & Folkman J. (2016). What great listeners actually do. Harvard Business Review. Accessed on December 7, 2022 at https://hbr.org/2016/07/what-great-listeners-actually-do.

PART II

APPLYING THE CONCEPTS

CHAPTER 7

Teaching Strength:
Practical Applications

I was talking to a client recently whose husband I also work with occasionally. While he is always perfectly pleasant while we are working together, I can never quite tell how much he gets out of our time. "How did he feel after I saw him Monday?" I asked.

"He is always in such a better mood when he comes in. I think he feels proud of himself, like he's accomplished something after being here."

In the next breath, she commented on how much she appreciates our work together. Earlier that week she had played golf with a couple of friends she hadn't seen for a while. They were unsteady on their feet and clearly not strong. "It just made me realize that the time I spend staying strong translates to other areas of my life."

As you have seen, different aspects of movement influence emotional health and well-being. One of the biggest causes of resistance to exercise, specifically strength training, that I have observed is a lack of accessibility. The exercises commonly portrayed or taught as beginner exercises don't always feel like an appropriate starting point for a true beginner. This makes people feel frustrated or like it's not a worthwhile pursuit.

Imagine that you are learning to play the piano. The first thing you will probably learn is where middle C is. Middle C is a home base on the piano and a common transition point.

Understanding common transition points is extremely helpful when someone is first approaching a strength program of any kind. It's like finding middle C—if you know how to be comfortable in a position that is the starting point or transition for many different movements, it gives you a sense of home base, a place you can always return to if something isn't working out (which happens whenever you learn something new). Home base can help you reset, find your sense of balance, and try again. We will explore the idea of common transition points in the exercises later in this chapter.

You will also be introduced to some of the more common causes of overuse injuries, such as tendinopathy and bursitis. Understanding different injuries can give you a more clear understanding of how to work with someone who is currently getting treatment from a medical professional for these injuries. It may also help you understand why experiencing these types of injuries can feel defining, as though the injury becomes the person, or how these injuries can lead to anxiety around moving in a way that causes the injury to recur.

At the end of the chapter you will find common strength-based exercises with key points to consider. This list is by no means exhaustive—once you understand basic concepts, the variations you can teach are limited only by your creativity—but they are good starting points for the exploration of strength.

But for now, let's talk about approaching a strength-training program, which is rather like approaching a blind date. You don't really know what to expect, but under the guidance of the right person or program, it can be good—really good. Creating the best first strength-training date for someone allows them to leave feeling like they accomplished something that could positively impact their life.

A baseline of basic strength makes all other movement feel more attainable. As you will see throughout this chapter, strength and mobility are not two separate entities. When taught thoughtfully, strength develops mobility and mobility develops strength. I mention this because if people are guarded or armored, holding themselves with an outer shell of rigidity that looks like it can't be penetrated, it could be argued that starting with strength is the wrong choice, that it will just add more stiffness and rigidity. This is only true if the person already has a regular basic strength-training routine (we will discuss this further in Chapter 8). Yes, it's absolutely true that there are people who are hypervigilant about their strength-training programs for external reasons or who perform it for an intrinsically motivated reason but don't have the variability or curiosity in their program to create range of motion in a variety of positions. As a result, they move stiffly and are not able to interact comfortably with the environment through movement despite being singularly strong and able to perform their regular exercises perfectly. I have witnessed the same thing in other modalities as well, watching as the Pilates practitioner or yoga teacher moves elegantly into an impressive position yet is unable to get up and down from the floor in a way that requires coordinated strength and mobility. Any time exercises are done repetitiously at the expense of exploring other ways to move, an individual's movement vocabulary becomes limited. When movement vocabularies are limited to a set repertoire of movements, the individual's ability to view the ways they can interact with the environment becomes more narrow. When it comes to movement, variety creates a more adaptable mindset that seeps into all aspects of well-being.

But the ability to move variably begins with strength, basic strength, the kind that lets someone pick up a box of books without being afraid they are going to injure themselves or that gives them a sense of center. "Wait," you might be thinking. "What about all of those people who get injured when they begin a strength-training program?"

Muscles get stronger when there is load placed upon them. They adapt and strengthen in order to withstand the increased demand on the system. When load exceeds the capacity to adapt, injury can occur. For instance, when the forces generated within muscles exceed the tendon's loading capacity, the tendon becomes injured (Brewer, 2017). This gets tricky because load is what creates adaptation, so you need to load things enough that adaptation can occur, but if you load things too much, the body rebels and tissues don't have time to get strong enough to withstand the new repeated stress of external load.

The way to avoid injury is to progress slowly, giving the musculoskeletal system adequate time to adapt and build the capacity to withstand greater forces.

"Fine," you might say. "What about the discomfort associated with loading?" This, too, is tricky, but as long as you begin with manageable progressions that feel safe, you will be okay.

Why do I keep talking about feeling safe? Neuroception, remember, is an unconscious perception of safety. The very nature of strength-based exercise is that there will be a SNS response. This isn't bad, but if the SNS response spirals into overdrive, that will alter how the person is moving and make them contract above and beyond what is needed to perform the movement. The most obvious example of this actually can be seen while stretching. If you try and move your leg into a position it hasn't been in since you were five, what happens?

Unless you are hypermobile, you contract away from the position as a complex interplay of excitatory responses occur, causing a muscular contraction in the very muscle you are attempting to stretch (Shemmell *et al.*, 2010). It's as though your brain says, "Danger! Danger! Unknown territory! Not safe!" The response is to signal the muscles to move away from the potentially dangerous situation. This isn't unlike what happens when you grab a hot pan, except that it happens not because the pan was unexpectedly hot; rather, it happens because you made a conscious choice to try something you weren't ready for. It's entirely possible that you will be able to get into the position in three months if you break the skill down and begin with a safe, basic progression, but that requires meeting yourself where you are.

And this is the biggest problem people run into when they begin a strength-training program. They begin where they think they should be, not in a place that supports their current ability while challenging them just enough. This, unfortunately, doesn't set people up for success; it sets them up for failure and potentially sets them up to stay away from weights altogether because they now believe they are dangerous or potentially harmful.

One of the roles of the coach or teacher is to lay foundations. If a coach is working with someone who wants to please them or is willing to work hard at home to make progress faster, an attuned coach will slow them down by giving them the appropriate progressions, reminding them that it's not about sets and reps, and not setting too much home-work because, unlike most people, this client will actually do more than is asked of them because they want to get there sooner (what sooner is, exactly, is an ambiguous point that could be the subject of another chapter).

As you move through this chapter, you may find yourself thinking the baseline progressions are too easy for most people. Many people who seek out the guidance of a teacher or coach lack basic strength; taking the time to develop the most fundamental aspects of strength will benefit these individuals tremendously and help them create the confidence they need to progress in a pain-free way.

A Brief Note about Nervous System Sensitivity

When you begin strength-based work with people who are extremely deconditioned or those who have a lot of fear around exercise, it's not uncommon for there to be a lot of initial nervous system sensitivity. For instance, if you are working with someone who has chronic low back pain and you place the person in a position that requires a minimal amount of load in the low back, they may still tell you they feel it in the low back. Using the tools you have developed through instructing and changing the individual's focus should redirect the sensation to something else, like their contact with the floor or the sensation of muscular work in a different area. Another option is to leave the position, do something else the person doesn't feel in the low back, and return to the initial position to see if they still feel sensation they equate with back pain. When the client performs an exercise that makes them feel strong and capable, it can change how they experience the previously uncomfortable position or movement because they feel successful and supported.

The thing with chronic pain is that it can co-exist with anxiety and/ or depression (Gong *et al.*, 2018). Respecting a client's concern regarding chronic pain while implementing thoughtful programming to improve the overall sense of strength can have a profound impact on overall well-being. Exercise isn't a panacea for symptoms related to mental health, but it is an important part of helping a person find physical and emotional balance.

What sensations, then, are cause for concern? Things like pinching or closed-angle joint pain are not sensations to push into. These types of sensations can indicate alterations in the bone, some of which may resolve with exercise and conservative treatment (Nakamura *et al.*, 2016). However, it's not your job to determine or diagnose why the sensation is occurring; it is your job to recognize what it looks like and know when to reroute.

So, what does closed-angle joint pain look like? If I come into a tall half kneeling position with my right foot forward and I shift my right knee and torso over my right ankle and there is pain on the front of the foot at the ankle joint, that is closed-angle pain. A stretching sensation in the back of the ankle or a sense of working in the front of the shin (which can happen, depending on how the movement is instructed) are appropriate sensations. Muscular effort feels different than a hard stop or joint pain.

You always have the option in these situations to slow the movement way down and make it quite a bit smaller. The smaller, slower movement decreases the sensation of risk and increases feelings of safety. This gives the client an opportunity to still feel like they are able to accomplish the original task at their own level. Though this is a mobility example and not a strength example, the principles remain the same.

For instance, if you ask your client to perform a deep squat (this is either a mobility exercise or strength-based exercise, depending on how it's taught) and they experience pinching in the front of the hip, you have several choices. You can change the foot position to see if that eliminates the discomfort. You can avoid the position altogether. You can have the person not go down as low, asking them to stop before the pinching begins. You can also step away from the squat, ask the person to perform two or three targeted hip exercises, create a sensation of work in the abdominals, and do an integrated foot-to-hip exercise. This type of movement intervention redirects attention, changes proprioception, and improves kinesthetic awareness of other areas. Once they have finished, you can ask them to try the squat again and see if anything changes.

All of these ways of approaching the sensation in the hip may be effective; the right option depends on the client and their needs. The goal is to create a sense of autonomy and strength. I tend to use avoidance as a last resort, preferring to see if I can find an alternative way of performing the movement that works, but that's just me. Play with different interventions and see what resonates most with you and, of course, with the person in front of you.

I have worked with a handful of people who have needed hip or knee replacements or had shoulder cysts, and the sensations they experience and how they move are very different than someone with non-specific chronic pain or an overly activated SNS. The beauty is you can still help someone get strong in the rest of their body so they feel strong and capable heading into surgery; you can also perform low-level mobility exercises in a pain-free range with minimal loading in the injured limb. Strength training isn't something to fear; it's something to celebrate and it can be taught in a way that honors a person's current physical state while still building up strength.

Bursitis

"But Jenn," you may be wondering, "what about more serious chronic injuries related specifically to tissue damage, like bursitis or tendinopathies?"

Bursae are small sacs lined with synovial fluid that provide a cushion between tendons and bones (Hirji *et al.*, 2011). They exist throughout the body at all of the major joints, including the shoulder, elbow, hip, knee, and ankle. When someone is diagnosed with bursitis, they are being diagnosed with inflammation of the bursae surrounding the joint (for the anatomy enthusiasts out there, "bursa" refers to a singular sac; "bursae" is the plural, referring to more than one sac).

Interestingly, research suggests that lateral hip pain, which for many years was believed to be caused by trochanteric bursitis, may actually be caused by gluteal tendinopathy or gluteal tears in up to 50 percent of reported cases (Reid, 2016). The exact mechanism for what causes the pain remains unclear. If you work with people in a one-on-one setting for long enough, the chances are high that, at some point, someone will arrive in obvious discomfort in a specific area with no obvious injurious or traumatic cause for the onset of pain. Understanding what some potential causes of discomfort look like makes it easier for you to create a movement program that works around the issue without making things worse and while still improving strength, mobility, and confidence in the rest of the body.

Greater trochanteric pain syndrome is characterized by chronic lateral hip pain that increases during active hip abduction, passive hip adduction, and direct pressure, like palpation or lying on the side that hurts (Lustenberger *et al.*, 2011; Speers & Bhogal, 2017). Fortunately, conservative treatment, including physical therapy and a thoughtful exercise program, leads to a resolution of symptoms in most subjects.

Tendinopathy

Tendons attach muscle to bone. Pain associated with tendon inflammation is called tendonitis; when there are degenerative changes in the tendon structure, it is called tendinosis. "Tendinopathy" is a term that has recently become associated with reduced tendon function and pain. The causes of tendinopathy are multifactorial and can result in chronic pain, weakness, and susceptibility to further injury (Lipman *et al.*, 2018). One important aspect of rehabilitation is exercise and load management, focusing at first on emphasizing targeted strength and control, followed by loaded strengthening.

Research suggests that the main goals of conservative treatment in conditions like greater trochanteric pain syndrome and tendinopathy are to manage load, reduce compressive forces across the affected joint, strengthen the muscles surrounding the joint, and treat any comorbid conditions. Initially, positions that cause pain should be avoided. Unless you are a physical therapist or physiotherapist, your job isn't to treat anything; however, you can successfully help clients manage load, build control, and strengthen the tissues around the joint in a pain-free manner.

Let's move on to some practical applications of these concepts. A great way to approach any strength-based exercise is through the steps applied in tendinopathy rehabilitation: manage load, initially emphasize targeted strength and control, and eventually use external load to get stronger.

Managing Load

In order to manage load effectively, it should be dispersed across the structures supporting the joint. One way to achieve this is through "co-contraction," the simultaneous contraction of the muscles surrounding the joint to maintain joint stability (Heitmann *et al.*, 2012). Co-contraction is essential for postural stability and is responsible for our ability to resist external perturbations (Kim & Hwang, 2018). Improving an individual's sense of co-contraction, then, will make them feel like they have more control, because joints feel more stable. Co-contraction also creates an overall sense of resilience. When your joints feel like they are supported by muscular strength, you feel less likely to be knocked over by external forces in the environment.

Remember in Chapter 6, when we discussed how movement happens and how it can occur consciously and unconsciously? If people have never thought about how their joints are supported or considered different ways to apply load across a limb, performing basic isometric contractions with specific attention to position and application of load makes the movement conscious. It disrupts habitual patterns, and because it is performed in a slow, safe manner, the emphasis is on the sensation of work rather than the conscious monitoring or whether or not there is a potential risk of injury associated with the movement.

EXERCISE: SEATED ISOMETRIC CONTRACTION

Let's revisit isometric contractions and play with the idea of co-contraction.

Come into a seated position on a chair. Find the connection points of the feet, focusing on the heels, the big-toe balls of the feet, and the pinkie-toe balls of the feet pressing into the ground.

Once you have the sensation of the feet pressing into the floor, begin pushing the floor away from you. Press so much that it feels as if you were about to stand up. Where do you feel the work? Hold there for three breaths.

Relax. Take a moment to rest. Begin pressing your feet into the floor again, but this time, imagine that the shins are shifting forward over the ankles. Notice how that changes how your feet are pressing into the ground. Hold for three breaths.

Rest for a moment. Imagine that you are reaching the pinkie-toe edges of the feet long. Maintain the sense that the pinkie-toe edges of the feet are reaching long as you press down into the floor, preparing to stand up. Hold this position for three breaths. Rest. How does that feel?

Now stand up and sit down three or four times. Does that feel easy or hard? Challenging or smooth?

There are several muscles that allow mobility, stability, and strength at the hip joint. It is not uncommon for people to be afraid that squatting will hurt their knees or to feel discomfort in their knees when they stand up or sit down. By managing load and teaching someone how to feel support through different areas of the body, you give them an opportunity to feel how the hip joint is supported by different muscles. This introduces variability of load across the joint and (usually) makes the joint feel more stable, translating into a more effortless transition to standing.

The instructions above emphasize creating stability or work in the anterior, medial, and lateral portion of the hips. Teaching the sensation of work in the posterior chain is also important. The hamstring muscle group connects the pelvis to the back of the knee, providing the sensation of support throughout the back side of the upper leg (Elias *et al.*, 2015).

EXERCISE: ISOMETRIC HIGH SQUAT

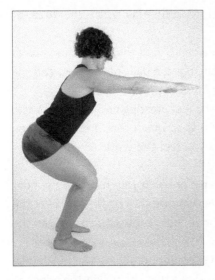

Come into a standing position with your feet a little more than hip distance apart and your toes in whatever position feels comfortable. Feel the feet against the floor, specifically the center of the heels, the big-toe balls of the feet, and the pinkie-toe balls of the feet. Move as if you were sitting back into a chair. When you get close to where you imagine the chair would be, hold that position.

Imagine that someone is trying to pull your hips down further towards the floor and you are resisting that person. Hold that position as the imaginary person tries to pull you down towards the floor for three breaths.

Relax back up into a standing position. How did that feel?

Now place your back against a wall and walk your feet forward so you are leaning your back and hips against the wall and your feet are pressing into the floor. Make sure your pelvis isn't tucked; if you had an imaginary tail, it would be pointing slightly backward, not between your legs.

Slide your hips down the wall until your knees are bent between 45 and 90 degrees. Make sure your feet are still pressing into the floor as if you were pushing it away and you feel the connection of the heels with the floor.

Imagine that someone is trying to pull your hips down the wall and you are resisting, not letting your hips slide at all. Imagine that the person pulling is fairly strong, so you have to work hard to resist.

Hold this position for three breaths. Straighten your legs and rest. How did that feel?

Imagining how to resist a force usually triggers the sensation of work in a three-dimensional way around the flexed joints without using any extra words. Once people understand how to do this in an isometric position, it's generally easy to translate into movement. As someone lowers down into a squat, for instance, if they imagine they are actively resisting a person who is pulling them into the position, they will generally feel both their quadriceps and their hamstrings working. This creates the sensation of stability and makes the work of the movement feel more evenly distributed.

How would you make the load variable in either of the last two exercises? The easiest way is by changing the foot position. There is no rule that says you have to learn how to load your hips with your feet in a specific position. If the position were loaded with an external object such as a weight, it's possible you would find individual preferences for foot position in order to maximize efficiency; even then, however, as people become stronger and more confident, altering the foot position changes the loading patterns throughout the legs. Obviously, you shouldn't try this if you are attempting to squat with the highest amount of weight possible, but if you are performing sub-maximal lifts, playing with foot position can actually open doors to more efficient positions that you might not have considered before; it will also increase your strength and tolerance to a variety of positions.

Other ways to vary load include changing torso position or arm position. Any subtle shift will change how load is dispersed through the structure, which means there are many ways to help someone feel work in different areas.

A Note on Torso Position

If someone initiates a squat at their low back instead of their hips, teaching the person how to feel a sense of center will both improve their sense of stability and help them feel what it's like to move from the hip versus the lumbar spine. There are two ways you can do this: by using an external task/constraint or by increasing awareness of the lumbar spine.

Using an external task or instruction gives the person a frame of reference for where the body is oriented in relation to the object. For instance, if someone arches their low back every time they squat even when I ask them if they can squat without arching their back and I give them an object with a bit of weight, like a sandbag, medicine ball, or kettlebell, how they squat will change. The additional weight limits the number of ways they can do the action of squatting and, depending on where the weight is held, will bias the movement so that there is less likelihood of the movement being initiated by arching the back. The extra weight both increases awareness of the position of the torso and changes the center of mass. Any time you change the center of mass, how a movement is performed will also change.

Another example of a constraint would be to change the foot position by placing the feet on a slanted surface with the toes lower than the heel. Changing the position of the feet will change the position of the torso (and changing the position of the torso will change the position of the feet).

When any movement task is performed, there are many ways the CNS could organize the joints to perform the movement. Each joint has multiple degrees of freedom, or options, for movement (Latash *et al.*, 2010). The introduction of the weight as a constraint changes the number of ways the squat can be performed and, more often than not, results in a more upright, connected torso. What I mean by connected is the ribs will move into a more downward and naturally oriented position to allow for the object to be held efficiently. If I introduce a breathing aspect to this task on top of the constraint, not only will the individual feel more stable and more aware of where the body is located in space, they may also feel a sensation of muscular work in the abdominals, increasing body awareness and interoceptive awareness.

Instead of adding weight or a slant board (or both), you could also have the person perform spinal mobility before squatting. For instance, you could use cat/cow variations, emphasizing lumbar and pelvic movement. Cat/cow can be performed several different ways. The most traditional version is to come into a quadruped position and round and arch the spine without rocking the torso forward or backward. The movement is purely up towards the ceiling and down towards the floor.

Teaching someone how to differentiate different aspects of the spine improves motor control and creates a more clear, conscious image of their body and how it moves in space. For instance, if you begin by asking the client to arch and round the spine a few times and then ask them to keep all of the spine still except for the lumbar spine, you will interrupt the habitual way they perform the task. This requires conscious effort to figure out how to move just the lumbar spine and can lead to an improvement in body schema and kinesthetic awareness. You could ask the client to move the pelvis or different parts of the thoracic spine instead of just moving the lumbar spine...you get the idea.

Once the client understands how to move the pelvis and lumbar spine in isolation, you can ask them to perform the squatting pattern again without moving the pelvis or lumbar spine. Because the client just spent time consciously moving the spine, it will have become easier to feel when the lumbar spine and pelvis are moving and, hypothetically, to move from the hips instead of the back.

Which choice is the right choice? It depends on the client. If the client is hypermobile and not very body aware, the more you can use constraints to limit movement options, the less frustrated the client will become, and, generally speaking, the less they will fixate on whether they are performing the movement in the right or wrong way. Because there are fewer ways to perform the movement, the reduction in choices enables the client to focus on the task (hold the external load and squat down) rather than worry about how they are squatting.

This is particularly valuable in hypermobile clients with fear or kinesiophobia associated with movement and exercise. Using fewer internally based instructions and more task-based activities allows the client to focus their attention on something other than their body. This gives their body a chance to self-organize without cognitive interruption, which is extremely useful, at least initially.

Conversely, for someone who lacks body awareness and doesn't have a clear mental image of their physical body, connecting to the body through conscious awareness can begin to create a sense of embodiment. In fact, sometimes just the act of feeling more of their physical body is enough to elicit a noticeable change in things like posture. Creating a mind/body connection can lead to an increased sense of safety, which downregulates the SNS, reducing excess muscular tone. (The same is actually true for the hypermobile client. It's almost like the sensation of muscular effort without the fear of injury gives them permission to trust that they are physically strong.)

EXERCISE: SPINAL MOBILITY

Come into a comfortable standing position. Observe your spine and where it's located in relation to your head, pelvis, and feet. Take a moment to feel which parts of you expand when you inhale and which parts contract when you exhale.

Gently nod your chin towards your chest. Lift the chin away from the chest. Do this three or four times.

Begin drawing a circle with your chin. Go two or three times in one direction and then go two or three times in the other direction. As you draw the circle, what happens if you keep the rest of the body still? Can you isolate the movement to the chin?

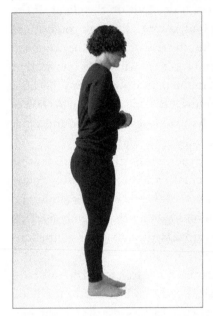

Place your hands on your ribs. Gently move the ribs back, away from the hands and then forward into the hands. Do this two or three times.

Pause for a moment. Keep your hands on the ribs as you draw a slow circle with the ribs. Go two or three times in one direction and two or three times in the other direction. What happens if you draw the circle while keeping the rest of the body quiet? What happens if you draw the circle without keeping the body quiet? How do these two conditions feel different?

Place your hands on your belly button. Move the belly button away from the hands. Move the belly button towards the hands. Do this two or three times.

Pause for a moment. Keep the hands on the belly button as you draw a slow circle with the belly button. Go two or three circles in one direction and two or three circles in the other direction. Can you draw circles while keeping the rest of the body quiet? Can you draw circles while letting the rest of the body respond? Which condition feels more challenging?

Imagine that you have a tail. Draw a line on the floor with your tail between your legs and behind you. Trace the line two or three times.

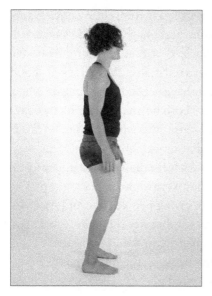 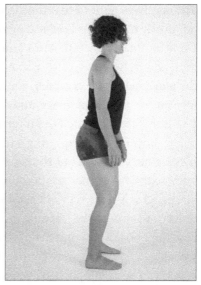

Pause. Draw a small circle on the floor with your tail, a medium circle on the floor with your tail, and a large circle on the floor with your tail. Repeat in the other direction.

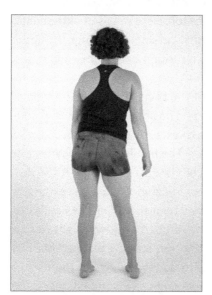 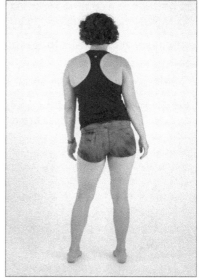

How much did the rest of your body move when you drew circles? Did the size of the circle affect how much the rest of your body moved?

You may have noticed that the directions I gave were clear, concise, and not overly text heavy. I did use metaphorical imagery when I suggested using an imaginary tail, and I emphasized primarily externally based focal points; however, I also asked you to self-reflect When I asked about the movement and how it felt, you may have needed to try it again while focusing on your experience, and that's both normal and perfectly okay. It's often difficult to focus on internal sensations when you are learning a new movement or exploring a familiar movement in a different way. It's also possible some of the sensations were dialed right up and you knew exactly how they felt because they were impossible to ignore. We discussed self-reflection in Chapter 6; giving people time and space to reflect assists with the learning process and makes them more aware of how their bodies respond to different instructions and positions. This is valuable for creating more connection between the mind and the body, which can be accomplished even in a strength-based scenario.

EXERCISE: QUADRUPED POSITION

The quadruped position, aka hands and knees position, aka prone table-top position, is a common starting place for strength-based movements. The ability to maintain a sense of strength and stability through the upper extremity makes it easier for people to transition away from—and return to—this position.

Before we begin, think about all of the things that need to happen for a person to even get into a quadruped position. What mobility concerns are there? What areas are prone to excessive sensation?

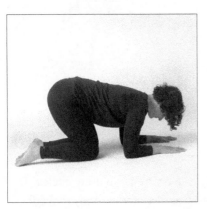

The number-one mobility concern is wrist extension. If the person lacks adequate wrist extension or strength, loading the hands in a quadruped position might not be the best starting place. What can you do instead (other than begin working on wrist mobility)?

You can shorten the lever arm by placing the person in a forearms and knees position instead. This

has the additional benefit of giving the person an opportunity to concentrate on controlling fewer joints. Shortening the lever arm reduces
the degree of freedom available because there are fewer joints involved.
This can make the position feel more accessible and/or approachable.

A quick side note: if someone is unable to place weight on the hands
when they are on a quadruped position on the floor, I will often work on
loading the hands in a position that requires less load, such as placing
the hands on a wall or on a high box. Most people are eventually able
to gain the mobility and strength needed to place the hands flat on the
floor comfortably. There are certain conditions, such as in the presence of arthritis that has altered the shape of the hands or Dupuytren's
contracture, a genetic disorder that causes flexion of the fingers and
significantly reduces range of motion, where a quadruped position or
straight-arm plank position on the floor might not be a good choice
for that individual. One of the coach's goals is to explore alternative
positions that don't require wrist extension (Sood *et al.*, 2013).

Other mobility concerns include the inability to straighten the
elbow (this can decrease the sense of stability and strength in the upper
extremity) and having limited ankle mobility, which makes it difficult
to place the top of the foot against the floor or to extend the foot and
place weight on the bottom of the toes. Solutions include teaching the
client how to straighten the elbows in an open-chain or less load bearing
position, working on ankle and foot mobility in different positions, and/
or elevating the knees on a blanket or bolster, decreasing the amount
of ankle mobility needed to place the foot in a comfortable position.

A huge aspect of working successfully with individuals who are experiencing symptoms related to anxiety, trauma, or depression is being
attuned to their comfort level and needs. The ability to identify factors
that may affect their success builds trust and shows clients that you
are paying attention. It also gives them an appropriate starting place.
With consistency, their mobility, strength, and tolerance to different
positions will increase. The starting position isn't a forever position,
and the changes that deconditioned individuals experience will be so
rapid that they will feel a sense of success as positions like a quadruped
position become more accessible.

Hypervigilant individuals who come to you with a laundry list of injuries from overuse and pushing hard without paying attention will feel a deeper sense of work than they are accustomed to from slowing down and establishing a good starting position. This sensation of work gives them an opportunity to feel something in a sustained way that, at least in my experience, allows them to recognize the value of regressing before they move forward.

A Brief Note about the Elbow

The upper arm and lower arm are not perfectly aligned in humans. The "carrying angle" refers to the angle between the ulna and the torso. Basically, when your arms are by your sides and your palms are facing forward, the natural position between the upper and lower arm is the carrying angle.

Research suggests that women have a slightly greater carrying angle than men and that there is variation within the sexes; this means that carrying angle, like most things related to anatomy, is varied (Adhikari *et al.*, 2017).

More extreme carrying angles may look like the elbow joint is hyper-extending, moving into injurious territory. Fortunately, the elbow is extremely stable, so an extended arm with an apparently hyperextended elbow is no more at risk of injury than an arm that doesn't appear to be hyperextending, unless force is applied that moves it beyond its normal range of motion (De Almeida *et al.*, 2017).

This means that if someone has the ability to straighten their arms to the point where it looks like the elbows are bending backward or hyper-extending, as long as there is structural integrity throughout the upper extremity and the individual can feel a sensation of work throughout the arm, it's nothing to worry about,

Practical Application: Quadruped Set-Up

Let's explore different ways to set up this position on the forearms before exploring the straight-arm position.

Come into a forearms and knees position with the elbows directly under the shoulders and the knees directly under the hips. Find a place where it feels like your ribs are parallel with the floor and your head is in line with your spine. Your eyes will be looking forward, slightly past your fingertips.

Begin pressing your forearms into the floor. Imagine that the thumb sides of the forearms are pressing as much as the pinkie sides of the forearms.

Now imagine that the back of the upper arms, from the inside of the armpits to the inside of the elbows, are reaching into the floor. Once you have done that, imagine that a line from the outside of each shoulder to the outside of each elbow is also reaching into the floor.

Maintain this position for four to six breaths, focusing on the forearms, the outside of the upper arms, and the inside of the upper arms all reaching into the floor. When you have finished, relax. What do you feel?

It's not uncommon for people to struggle with maintaining integrity in the shoulder joint in this position. If you notice that the person you are working with is unable to reach through the back of the arms, it looks like the upper arms are rotating forward, or it looks like the shoulders are moving up towards the neck, you can play with instructing different arm actions. What you choose depends on what the person needs. How could you do this?

You can use your words or props. Let's imagine you want to use your words and the person needs more humeral adduction. If the person is on a yoga mat, you could ask them to get the sense that the elbows are gently pulling the yoga mat together. Or, if you have a half foam roller or a yoga block that is the appropriate width for the person (not too narrow), you could place the object between their elbows and ask them to gently press their elbows into the object. Which is likely to be more effective? Probably pressing the elbows into the yoga block. Why? Because the object provides tactile feedback. This allows the person to actually experience the action of pulling their arms towards midline; experiencing the desired action in a tangible way through an action-based focus reduces the chance the individual will worry about whether they are performing it correctly or utilize an unusual strategy by trying to fire specific muscles. The object acts like a constraint; constraints reduce degrees of freedom (Ito & Tsuji, 1992).

Another way to say this is that constraints reduce the number of ways a person will perform a task, especially if the constraint provides a clear path to action for the client to try. Once the individual learns how to produce the desired action with the object, it becomes easier to replicate the action without the object, because a frame of reference has been established.

Let's pretend the person doesn't understand how to rotate the upper arm out. What could you do? You could use your words and ask the person to gently pull the hands away from each other, causing a subtle external rotation action in the shoulder joint. You could also place a strap of some kind around the person's wrists and ask them to gently press out against the band or strap (such as a looped stretchy band of light/medium resistance or a yoga strap). You could also pause, use a basic awareness exercise to teach the person what external rotation feels like, and return to the movement after they understand the action you are looking for at the shoulder.

Or, if the person really understands how to do internal rotation at the upper arm, you could ask them to do more internal rotation of the upper arm and then go in the opposite direction. This gives the person a chance to contrast what is familiar with what is less familiar.

Which is the best choice? As always, it depends. The general rule of thumb is the more mobility a person has, the more they will benefit from physical constraints, like a strap or band. The more stiff a person is, the more likely they are to try and overpower the band or strap, which might make the verbal instruction of gently pulling the mat apart or an awareness/motor-control drill a potentially better choice.

What happens if the person feels the action in the neck? You need to make a change. You could alter the rib position, alter the neck position, ask the person to not use so much effort, or change the loading in the arms by shifting the torso back or performing the same action stand-ing against the wall. Once the person understands how to achieve the action in a position where there is less loading in the arms, try again in a more traditional quadruped position, either later in the session or the next time you see the person. Learning happens, remember, during the in-between times as much as it does in the moment. Giving people time to process sets them up for success later.

Optimal Duration for Isometric Contractions

How long should the person hold the isometric contraction? (All of these questions! But spending time thinking about the minute details prepares you to think critically and figure out what needs to happen for the client to be successful; it will also give you options for ways to help a client work through frustration or resistance to a specific concept.)

As with most things, it depends on what you are trying to accomplish and the client's personality. Isometric contractions can be performed at varying percentages of maximal voluntary contraction (MVC). If you ask someone to perform an isometric contraction at a low percentage of MVC, it may feel more approachable if the contraction is held for a longer duration. Conversely, if you ask someone to hold an isometric contraction while working at a high percentage of MVC, longer-duration holds will likely feel more challenging and possibly harder to maintain, appealing to people who like the sensation of work.

When researchers asked subjects to perform an isometric hand-grip task, they noticed that once subjects found a strong grip, it wasn't difficult to maintain force. The task was purposefully designed to prevent fatigue in the subjects, but interestingly, while it may have initially felt challenging to achieve the desired strength of grip, keeping it was less of a challenge (Pakenham *et al.*, 2020).

This makes sense from both a physiological and psychological level. Once your brain understands what needs to happen in the PNS to accomplish a task, it's easier to keep the signals (i.e., motor neurons) firing until fatigue sets in (fatigue, remember, can be caused by a number of things).

In a similar way, when you are initially exposed to something that feels really hard and you are able to accomplish it successfully, the experience becomes slightly less hard the next time you do it.

I use this concept regularly with a client who happens to have Parkinson's. Her tremor is pronounced in her right hand. Before she actually begins moving weighted objects, I have her hold the weights and do movements with the legs. It gives her nervous system a chance to establish how much force is needed to hold the weight. Once she has that, it's easy to move the weight in different positions. The tremor is still there, but for a moment, a connection is made between the CNS and the PNS.

Low-level isometric contractions can be a useful way to establish proprioception and help someone develop kinesthetic awareness of a specific area. Higher-level isometric contractions are useful for strengthening muscles and tendons in a specific position. During isometric contractions, sarcomeres are positioned in a fairly uniform way. Sarcomeres are the contractile units of a muscle fiber and are made up of actin and myosin. Actin and myosin are the active structures that are responsible for muscular contraction. When you isometrically contract a muscle in a position that feels weak or unstable, the sarcomeres line up and become stronger, hypothetically making the muscle stronger and able to tolerate more load in that specific position (Herzog *et al.*, 2015; Jackson & Neumann, 2019).

In research that looks specifically at increasing tendon stiffness, longer-duration isometric holds appear to be more effective for increasing tendon stiffness than shorter-duration holds (Kubo *et al.*, 2001). Tendons attach muscle to bone, and the elasticity of the tendon can be altered with physical training. Muscle fibers exert force that stretches the tendon before the force is transmitted to the bone. Tendon stiffness is believed to affect the amount of force a muscle can generate—the greater the tendon stiffness, the higher the amount of force generated (*ibid.*; Osawa *et al.*, 2018).

In our basic example of the quadruped position, holding the position with specific focal points is an isometric contraction at a lower level. This (hopefully) improves general awareness of the position of the body. It also allows the person an opportunity to feel different sensations associated with various set-ups. Asking the person to apply gentle pressure against the strap or band and then relax three or four times will allow them to feel the actions and internalize them, giving the nervous system an opportunity to approach what may be a potentially new position and figure out how to perform the action in a way that feels safe and controlled. It also opens a conversation between the coach and the client. If the client doesn't like the way a particular version feels or if they stumble across a variation that seems to work better for them, they have space to share and explore. There is no right or wrong way to experience a position; as a result, approaching different positions with curiosity and interest generally leads to a more enjoyable outcome (for both the client and the coach).

Once the person understands how to set up in a quadruped position, you can work on things like scapular retraction and protraction, crawling, quadruped rock backs... The possibilities are endless, and if you instruct things like reaching the elbow into the ground if the person you are working with is on their elbows, reaching the center heel of the palms into the ground if they are on their hands and knees, or reaching the knees into the floor, they will continue to find a sense of awareness and connection throughout their structure.

EXERCISE: HANDS AND KNEES FROM THE PERSPECTIVE OF THE UPPER BODY

Come onto a quadruped position, with your hands under your shoulders, or slightly forward if there's too much pressure on your wrists, and your knees under your hips. Begin reaching the center heels of the palms and all five fingertips of each hand into the floor. Imagine that there are two lines running parallel to each other on each arm from the inside armpit to the thumb and from the center of the outside of the shoulder to the pinkie. Reach those lines are long as you can. Make sure you are breathing. Hold this for four to six breaths. How does it feel?

Things to look for:

- Do the ribs stay parallel with the floor, or does the back arch or round?
- Do the index fingers rotate towards each other, do they point straight ahead, or do they point away from each other?
- Do the elbows look hyperextended?
- Is the person able to fully straighten the elbows?

These are simply observation points. They give you a frame of reference for potential habits, and some of these observations, like whether the elbows appear to be hyperextended, aren't things to change. They are visual information that can help you stay curious about how a person moves and their habits.

EXERCISE: HANDS AND KNEES FROM THE PERSPECTIVE OF THE LOWER BODY

Come into a quadruped position with your knees roughly under your hips and your hands roughly under your shoulders. Begin reaching the knees into the ground, as though the fronts of the thighs were getting long.

Keep the action of reaching the knees into the ground but see if you can make the back of the upper legs long as well. How does that feel?

Walk your knees back slightly behind your hips. Perform the same action of reaching the knees down, imagining the front and back of the thighs are getting long.

Finally, walk your knees forward of your hips a little but move them further away from each, so they are slightly outside of your hips rather than in the same line as your hips. Reach the knees down. How does that feel?

Things to look for:

- When the person reaches the knees down, does the pelvis shift?
- Does the person look down as they are reaching the knees into the ground?
- Which knee position did the client feel was easiest?
- Did the client feel one knee position was more supportive than another?

Again, these are just ideas, designed to pique your curiosity about different ways you can explore a basic transitionary position.

Once the person finds a quadruped position that feels supportive for them, if you want to add more load you can ask them to do things like float the knees off the floor, shift the hips back and forth, or crawl. You can add variation by altering the hand position, altering the body position (think an inverted "V" or down dog position), altering the foot position, shifting weight from side to side, or reaching one hand in different directions while leaving the other hand on the ground. All of these variations, if introduced thoughtfully, improve confidence and strength while creating a sense of stability in the quadruped position.

We have already discussed the fact that movement occurs throughout the brain. The planning and execution of voluntary motor movements occurs in both sides of the brain. A seemingly simple action like raising the left arm results in activation in the motor cortex in both the right and left sides of the brain (interestingly, research suggests that the dominant brain hemisphere is associated with controlling movement dynamics and trajectory control of both arms (Bundy *et al.*,

2018). Whether bilateral limb training or unilateral limb training is more effective depends on the goal of the movement program—in research on chronic stroke patients, bilateral arm training led to a reduction in impaired limb movement time and increased functional limb ability (Summers *et al.*, 2007). It has been suggested that bilateral arm movements engage additional brain circuits in the supplementary motor area and primary motor cortex over and above single-arm training movements, though a randomized controlled trial performed on stroke patients that compared bilateral arm training with auditory cueing[1] to unilateral limb training using development positions concluded that the two types of training led to different brain responses through different mechanisms (*ibid.*). A combination of both types of training may be ideal from a neurological standpoint.

Movements like shoulder abduction can sometimes feel more complex (meaning the client performs them in a less automated way) because they are performed less frequently than, say, reaching the arm over the head. These types of movements can challenge proprioception and kinesthetic awareness if they feel unfamiliar or awkward. Incorporating upper-extremity movements in a variety of positions has several benefits. Reaching out to the side requires a different stabilization strategy through the torso than reaching directly overhead. This introduces variability for the neuromuscular system. It also enhances the individual's mental image of their body and how it moves in space (Lee *et al.*, 2012; Brun *et al.*, 2019).

When you cross midline and move limbs into different parts of space where other limbs usually reside, the cognitive complexity increases. "Cross-lateral integration" is a term that is often used to describe an individual's ability to move the limbs across the body. It is a developmental milestone that is accomplished by the time children turn eight or nine years old and is implicated in body schema development and bilateral coordination (Lombardi *et al.*, 2000). Using positions like the quadruped position as a starting point to work with different arm movements and reaching patterns not only strengthens the body, it also challenges the brain.

---

[1] Auditory cueing means movements were performed at a set speed based on a metronome—the sound of the metronome is a cue to perform a certain action (Whitall *et al.*, 2011).

Practical Application: Hinge Position

The hinge position is a way to teach differentiation between the hip and the pelvis/low back. When loaded, it's also a great way to increase strength in the posterior chain, specifically the hamstrings, gluteal muscles, and torso (Andersen *et al.*, 2019).

Before we get into the actual position, think about the things you usually see when teaching people how to hip hinge. What are the common sticking points?

Difficulty shifting weight behind the ankles, an unclear understanding of how to move at the hips versus the pelvis, and a lack of strength in the torso all affect the ability to initiate a hip shift. If the person you are working with has strong postural habits, like a tendency to keep their pelvis forward and tucked under, hip hinging will be more challenging to teach. Why? From a motor control perspective, it may be as simple as the person not understanding how to move the pelvis behind the heels. In this case, teaching the action of moving the pelvis back first will make it easier to teach hip hinging. Instead of trying to teach someone who habitually thrusts their pelvis forward to move into a position that requires the management of multiple degrees of freedom (because there are multiple joints involved), take five minutes to teach them in a less complex position how to: a) move the pelvis and b) move the hips.

It's worthwhile to note that the pelvis can be an interesting place of tension and a difficult place to move from, especially if someone has experienced sexual trauma. If it is obvious that drawing focus to the pelvis is causing emotional distress and you are not a licensed therapist or psychologist, make sure you have a network of mental healthcare professionals to refer out to. When someone appears disconnected from an area like the pelvis, a therapist who specializes in somatic psychotherapy may be a good choice.

Assuming the pelvis isn't causing any emotional triggering when you draw attention to it, if you spend time teaching the client how to move the pelvis in different positions, it will be easier for them to feel: a) when the pelvis is moving and b) when the pelvis is remaining still.

Take a moment to think about the different positions you can ask someone to perform pelvic tilts in. How many did you come up with? The positions include: a supine position, prone quadruped position, prone position, tall kneeling position, seated position, half kneeling position, standing position, squat position, sumo squat position, split stance position, staggered feet position, seated long sit position, seated butterfly position... The options are endless. Which is the position that will be easiest for most people to grasp?

Usually, it's the supine position with knees bent and feet flat on the floor because it offers the most feedback. The brain loves feedback regarding position—feedback provides information about whether the task is being accomplished in the desired way. The feedback loop creates an opportunity for learning.

Sometimes, the person can't get the action of a pelvic tilt when supine because they are trying too hard or searching for too much feedback from the floor. When this happens, you can easily reroute by performing pelvic tilts seated, in a tall kneeling position, in a half kneeling position, or standing. Don't be afraid to veer off course and give your client (and yourself) space to try things out to see what resonates.

Let's say someone experiences discomfort in their low back while performing pelvic tilts. What should you do then? You should ask the person to make the movement smaller or imagine what it would be like to perform the movement in a pain-free way. Though there are times when the lumbar spine doesn't tolerate pelvic movement, in my experience, most people can regain movement in this area if they start small or spend time visualizing the action.

Why? Because of motor imagery. Motor imagery causes activation in the areas of the brain that are involved in movement preparation and execution. Lighting up these parts of the brain through imagination may facilitate motor learning when you perform the skill in real life (Mulder, 2007). Often, one of the reasons people experience discomfort during pelvic tilts is because they are bracing in other parts of the body. Visualization can help someone to observe where they grip or brace and to imagine what it would be like to not grip or brace. (Slowing down and/or moving slowly can also be useful for helping people identify unconscious movement habits.)

How many pelvic tilts should someone do? Usually one to two sets of four to eight repetitions is sufficient for the client to feel what it's like when the pelvis moves. If you follow up pelvic tilts by keeping the pelvis still, this often translates well into standing positions. For instance, if I ask someone to perform supine pelvic tilts and then ask them to keep the pelvis still while marching the feet in place, they will begin to understand how to consciously control the pelvis by letting it move and how to keep the pelvis still while the legs move around it.

Once you establish awareness, it's often easier to teach things like the hip-hinging pattern. We know that removing tactile feedback makes it more difficult to understand how the body is moving in space; ergo, adding tactile feedback makes it easier to feel how the body is moving in space. While teaching hip hinging, adding tactile feedback may mean placing a dowel along the length of the spine and maintaining contact points with the head, back of the ribs, and bottom of the sacrum while the pelvis moves back. Or, if someone is having a difficult time holding the dowel behind their body and/or instructing the person to pay attention to the back of the body isn't working, it might mean placing a resistance band around the front of the pelvis and letting the band pull the pelvis back. Or perhaps it means having the person stand facing away from a wall and asking them to stick their butt out until it touches the wall. All of these are perfectly reasonable options for teaching hip hinging. They can be performed in tall kneeling or standing. Sometimes, adding a light load to hold in front of the chest, like a medicine ball or kettlebell, can provide enough feedback to allow the individual to feel movement in the spine, making it easier to move from the hips.

When you are teaching the hinge position in standing, it's important to ensure the client is connected to their feet. Since the feet are the client's only reference point for the ground, the more the client feels the feet and is able to experience them as a place of strength and support, the more likely they will be able to access the movement in an easeful way.

Another way to improve a sense of confidence in the position is to ask the client to hold the hinge position for three or four breaths. Not only does this cause an isometric contraction in the muscles that support the bottom of the hinge, it also gives the CNS a chance to get accustomed to staying there a little while.

We fear what we don't know. This is aggravated by predisposed ideas someone may have regarding bending and backs. When I first expose people to hip hinging, it is not uncommon for them to tell me, "But I thought bending was bad for my back?" If someone moves in and out of the position a few times safely and then holds the position and feels work, not pain, their perceptions about what they are capable of begin to shift, and when perceptions shift, so, too, does a person's belief in their capabilities.

Pulling

Just like the legs are capable of pushing and pulling, the arms are also capable of pushing and pulling. Learning to pull with the arms not only makes you stronger, it also creates a sense of stability throughout the shoulder joint. If you never practice pulling, your movement options in your upper body will decrease.

Because pulling isn't a movement that modern-day daily life requires very often, it isn't uncommon for people to not understand how to coordinate the upper extremity during pulling movements. Considering that shoulder pain affects 18–26 percent of adults at any given time, it shouldn't be surprising that people have a difficult time accessing movement—and strength—in different parts of the shoulder (Linaker & Walker-Bone, 2015).

What has to happen in order to pull the arms back?

TRY THIS: Come into a comfortable, supported standing position (by supported, I just mean your feel are connecting firmly to the floor and you feel grounded). Reach your hands out in front of you as though you were grabbing something. Now make strong fists and pull your arms back towards your body, allowing the elbows to move past the torso. What happens to your shoulders as the arms are pulled back? What happens to the shoulder blades?

As the elbows move past the torso, the shoulders begin to move back and the shoulder blades move back (retract). Because the shoulder girdle is a complex structure that includes the clavicle (collarbone), humerus (upper arm bone), and scapula (shoulder blade), when one area moves, it impacts joints throughout the entire kinetic chain. Another way of thinking about this is: movement in one area causes movement in another area.

What happens if the shoulders and shoulder blades don't move back? Just like with the pelvis, this might mean the person doesn't know how to retract the shoulder blades, externally rotate the shoulder (which is what happens when the shoulders move back), or both. What are your options?

You could teach the person how to move the shoulders and how to move the shoulder blades independently. Once the person understands how to perform these two pieces, it will be easier to integrate the shoulder and shoulder blade movement without needing to over-instruct.

What is the easiest way to do this? You can increase the tactile feedback. If you want the individual to feel the action of the shoulder and shoulder blade movement, teaching it in a supported position that feels safe will give them a clearer image of what it feels like to move the shoulders.

Supported Shoulder Awareness

Come into standing position with your back and pelvis resting against a wall and arms long by the sides of your body. Your palms will be facing your body. Turn the palms so they face out, away from the wall. Hold for a moment and return the palms to the starting position. Do this three or four times slowly. What direction do the shoulders move in when you rotate the palms away from the wall towards the front of the room?

In coordinated movement, as the palms rotate forward, the shoulders begin to move back towards the wall. If this doesn't happen because you only rotate at the elbow joint, initiate the movement by reaching the shoulders gently towards the wall as the palms rotate out. Perform that movement a few times and then return to the movement of rotating the hands. See if there is an increased sense of the shoulders moving back towards the wall as the palms rotate forward.

Once that is clear, you can play with the idea of retracting and protracting the shoulder blades by moving the scapulae together and apart while leaning against the wall. The head doesn't need to be against the wall—the wall serves as a barrier to prevent excessive movement through the torso. Do this three or four times. As you bring your shoulder blades together, in what direction do the shoulders move? As you bring the shoulder blades apart, in what direction do the shoulders move?

When you bring the shoulder blades together, the shoulders move backward, towards the wall. When you bring the shoulder blades apart, the shoulders move forward, away from the wall. If you add the action of the arms reaching forward, grabbing tightly on to something, and pulling back, there should be a sense of integration of the shoulders moving towards the wall and the shoulder blades moving towards each other as the elbows move past the body. As the arms reach forward, you should eventually feel the shoulders moving forward and the shoulder blades moving away from each other.

What happens if someone feels this action in the low back? What is a common coordination sticking point? The answer is rib position. In this particular movement variation, even though the shoulder blades are moving, the spinal column is staying relatively still. If you notice the ribs flaring forward and up as someone moves the elbows past the body, a simple way to explore this is to ask them to move their ribs a few times, move the ribs while moving the arms, and move the arms without moving the ribs. Drawing attention to the feeling of the ribs moving (or not) as the shoulder blades move gives the client a choice: does it increase the efficiency during this particular exercise to move the ribs? Does it feel different if I don't move the ribs? What feels better for my low back when I pull my arms back: rib movement or no rib movement?

The best movement efficiency and coordination depends on the individual and what they are doing. There are times, like when you are performing a muscle-up, when a rib flare as you pull up makes sense. There are also times, like during a basic cable row, when flaring the ribs during scapular retraction isn't going to make things more efficient or coordinated in any way for the average person who just wants to work on basic horizontal pulling.

Some more examples of how to help someone feel their ribs can be found below.

EXERCISE: SUPINE RIB MOVEMENT

Come onto your back with your knees bent and your feet flat on the floor. Place your hands on the lower portion of your ribs. Gently guide your ribs towards the floor as you exhale. As you inhale, gently relax the ribs away from the floor. Go back and forth between these positions three or four times. On your last one, keep the ribs towards the floor as you inhale. Exhale, maintain the position or guide the ribs even closer to the floor. Repeat for three breaths. What do you feel happening in your ribs?

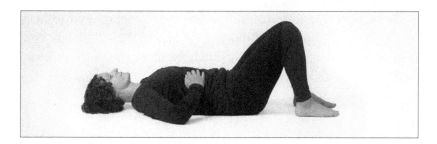

You might wonder why you'd use the breath, as I said earlier that drawing attention to the breath might increase anxiety. The ribs are designed to move in a three-dimensional way when you breathe, expanding on the inhale and contracting on the exhale. This particular exercise sequence highlights the physical response the body has to breathing. Because the breath causes an action that can facilitate body awareness and improve proprioception, it's worthwhile exploring it in positions like this. Additionally, using the breath to create movement rather than trying to control the breath can make breath work more accessible.

EXERCISE: USING A STRAP FOR FEEDBACK

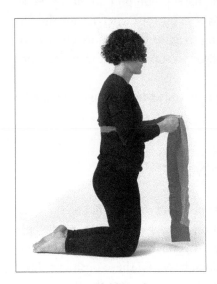

Come into a seated position on a chair holding a yoga strap or resistance band. Place the strap or band around the lower ribs and hold the taut strap in front of you. As you exhale, gently push the back ribs into the strap, attempting to move the strap backwards. As you inhale, move the back ribs forward, away from the strap. Do this three or four times, holding on the last one, attempting to push the strap further behind you for two or three breaths.

"But wait," you might be wondering. "What about thoracic extension and thoracic rotation?"

Remember, this intervention is specifically being used to help someone feel the opposite of thoracic extension. We will discuss how to improve awareness and mobility in different aspects of the thoracic spine when we discuss mobility in Chapter 8.

Pulling the Arms Down

It is possible to pull the arms towards the body in a variety of orientations (or, as you will see, the body towards the arms). When your arms are extended straight out in front of your body, you are pulling the arms towards you horizontally, but when your arms are overhead, there is a more vertical pulling action. Horizontal pulling is what happens when you pull a door open; vertical pulling is what happens when you pull a bag down from the overhead compartment or you pull yourself up onto a counter (a regular occurrence when you are five foot one).

EXERCISE: PULLING DOWN

Come into a seated position. Make sure you can feel your sitting bones against the surface on which you are sitting and your feet on the floor (if applicable). These are your points of reference, or grounding points.

Reach your arms up, as though your hands were going to touch the ceiling. The palms can be facing whatever direction feels most comfortable for your shoulders.

As you exhale, make strong fists and pull the elbows by the side of the body. Inhale, straighten the arms towards the ceiling, and open the hands.

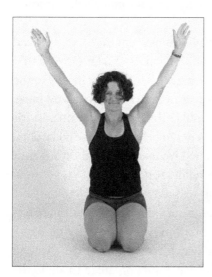
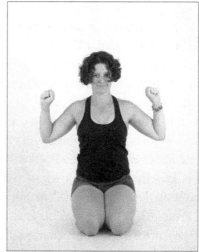

Perform this movement four times. What do you feel? And how do your shoulders move throughout the movement?

If you are struggling with feeling the actions of the arms and shoulders in this position, hold a dowel or resistance band. See if that makes the movement feel more clear.

As the hands and elbows move down, the shoulders move down. This becomes important when you are helping someone understand how to generate the force needed to pull the body up in a pull-up or pull the body forward in a crawling variation. When the hands are generating force in a specific direction, the arms follow, just like when the feet generate force in a specific direction, the hips follow.

For most of us, daily life doesn't require the arms to be overhead very often, and when we don't use specific movements regularly, it's easy to forget how many ways there are to reach the arms overhead.

If someone is fearful of taking the arms overhead or they simply haven't done it in years, it's not uncommon for areas near the shoulder to facilitate the overhead movement of the arms instead of the joints that make up the shoulder joint.

If you are interested in shoulder joint mechanics, you might want to know which four joints allow the arm to move in all the ways. They are the glenohumeral joint, scapulothoracic joint, acromioclavicular joint, and sternoclavicular joint.

Interestingly, another barrier for full extension of the arms overhead is linked to scapular kinematics. "Joint kinematics" is a fancy word that means how a joint moves. Scapular kinematics refers specifically to the ability of the scapula to abduct (move away from each other) and move up. As the arm goes overhead, the scapula rotates upwards and posteriorly tilts on the back of the rib cage. When this happens, the collarbone moves up and back. This results in effective load dispersal throughout the upper extremity (Ludewig & Reynolds, 2009).

Exactly how and how much the scapula rotates in a move like a pull-up depends on both the individual and the position of the hands (Prinold & Bull, 2016). This is true of all movements—varying hand, foot, or torso position changes the way force is distributed through the body. Variation also changes the way joints organize to allow the movement to occur.

I hope you are beginning to notice that teaching someone the foundations of a movement is most successful when the person feels like it is okay to try different things, there is some sort of tactile feedback regarding position, and there is space to reflect on the experience. As we discussed in Chapter 4, reflection is achieved by asking the person what they notice or feel and is a critical component both to increasing overall awareness and to learning.

EXERCISE: SHOULDER FLEXION WITHOUT RIB EXTENSION

Lean against a wall. Place your left hand on your lower right ribs. Your right arm will be long by the side of your body.

Exhale, reach the right arm up overhead. Use the left hand to help guide the right ribs back towards the wall as the arm goes overhead. Inhale, and lower the right arm back down.

Perform this four to six times, changing the position for the right palm each time so that it faces across the body, towards the body, and away from the body. Keep the eyes looking out as the arm reaches up and down. On the last one, hold the reaching position for two to three breaths, actively reaching the hand towards the ceiling. Rest, observing how you feel. Switch sides and repeat the movements.

After you have finished reaching the left arm, take a moment to compare the way the left and right arm felt. Was one side easier than the other? Why did it feel easier? Did one side feel stronger than the other?

To reduce the amount of perceived effort, you can perform this in a supine position on the floor using the floor as feedback for your back and torso. You can also add variability by reaching different places overhead, such as further away from midline or across the midline.

Once you have completed the last exercise, return to the original action of reaching the arms up and actively pulling them down. Does the movement make more sense?

EXERCISE: ACTIVE PULLING IN QUADRUPED

For this exercise, you will need a blanket and a floor on which the blanket will slide (like hardwood or laminate).

Come into a quadruped position with your hands on the blanket. Begin with your hands in front of your shoulders and your knees under your hips. Adjust your head so your eyes are looking towards your fingers and your ribs are lifting away from the floor.

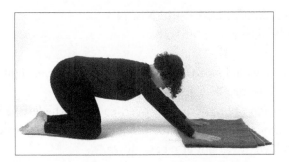

Actively pull the hands towards the knees. What happens? The blanket slides towards the knees. Reach the blanket back out to the starting position and repeat the action. Perform this four to six times. What has to happen in order for this to occur?

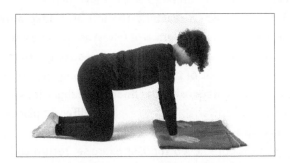

EXERCISE: ACTIVE PULLING IN SEATED

For this exercise, you will need a vertical object of some sort. You can use the corner of a rig in the gym, a pole like I am using here, or the corner of a swing set. (For simplicity's sake, the directions say "pole," but really, you can use any sturdy vertical object.)

Come into a seated position facing the pole. Place the soles of the feet against the pole (the knees will split away from each other, coming into a butterfly position). Reach the hands up, taking hold of the pole with the arms straight. One hand will be higher than the other.

Pull the pole down in the direction of the hips with the top hand. Remove the bottom hand from the pole and place it above the top hand. Hold for a count of three and then repeat, pulling with the top hand as you remove the bottom hand and place it above the top hand.

Walk your hands up three or four times, pulling as you walk the hands up and pulling as you walk the hands down. The hips will come off the floor as you walk the hands up.

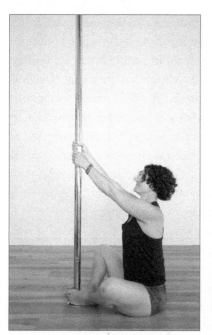 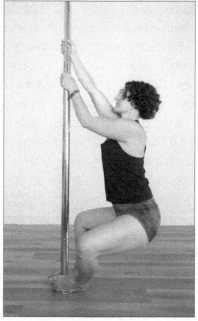

Some people will find that as soon as they begin actively pulling down, the hips will lift off the floor. Others will have difficulty figuring out how to generate the pulling action. When the hands begin to actively pull the pole, the shoulders and ribs will subtly move down. The more the person is able to grasp the pole with all of the fingers, including the pinkie fingers, the more they will be able to co-contract throughout the upper extremity and torso.

This relates to motor irradiation, an idea put forth by Sir Charles Sherrington that says when a muscle contracts, the contraction spreads to neighboring areas based on duration and intensity (Nunes *et al.*, 2016). This means that the more of yourself you can use to manage load, the more you will be able to do things like generate enough force to move the body.

The exercises below are variations on all of the themes discussed above. Focused strength can be taught in any joint; I have chosen to focus on four basic compound movements everyone can benefit from in these exercises, but you can apply the principles of basic strength for any strength-based skill.

Each variation is followed by bullet points with examples of where attention can be focused. The variations are by no means exhaustive; after you teach clients how to generate force and feel the parts of themselves that contribute to various aspects of movement, you are limited only by your creativity. It's worthwhile to note that once clients understand and can feel their bodies, you don't need to instruct throughout the exercise; in fact, for learning purposes, it can be really beneficial to ask the client afterwards, "Did you notice you rolled to the outside of your left foot while you were squatting? Next time, can you try keeping the big-toe side of the foot down, too?" This not only gives the client an opportunity to reflect and ponder how they were performing the skill, it also respects their intelligence and gives them choice.

Though I have never had anyone say, "No, I can't do that," giving them permission to try something and see if it works increases autonomy and, over time, makes them less reliant on you to tell them they are performing an exercise correctly—they will be able to feel how they are performing the exercise and self-correct to make things more efficient. Empowering people to trust their abilities to feel and perform strength-based movements translates beyond the walls of a gym.

Pushing Examples

Below are some exercise that explore the act of pushing in the upper body. This is where all of the time we spent on the foundational set-up of the quadruped position will make sense.

EXERCISE: HANDS AND KNEES TO KNEELING PRONE POSITION

Begin in a tall kneeling position or sitting on your heels, whichever feels more comfortable. Place your hands on the floor and walk your hands forward until you can lower down to your stomach. Push yourself back up away from the floor and walk your hands back to the tall kneeling or seated position.

Things to look for:

- Do the elbows bend?
- Do you lower down and press up evenly, or do you favor one side over the other?
- Are you breathing?

EXERCISE: PLANK TO DOWN DOG

Begin in a straight-arm push-up position. (You can do this with your hands elevated on a chair or table if you aren't comfortable in a straight-arm push-up position on the floor.)

Keep your arms straight as you push the hands into the floor and forward, letting your hips shift back to down dog. Use your hands to pull you back forward into a plank. Go back and forth four to six times.

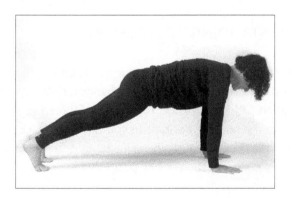

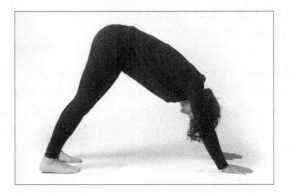

Things to look for:

- Can you keep the ribs lifted away from the floor?
- Do you tense your jaw?
- Can you actually shift the hips up and back, or are you tucking the pelvis to do the movement? (If you are tucking the pelvis, bend the knees when you shift the hips back.)
- Are you breathing?

If this movement feels relatively easy, when you shift back to down dog, lift the left hand off the floor and touch the right knee. Lower the left hand back to the floor as you rock forward to plank and then switch sides. This requires more balance, stability, and strength through the torso.

EXERCISE: STANDING TO A PUSH-UP

Begin in a standing position. Place your hands on the floor with your fingers pointing straight ahead. Walk the hands forward until you are in a plank position. Either pause here for a count of three and then walk the hands back to the starting position so you can stand back up, or lower yourself down to the floor, push yourself back up to a plank position, and walk your hands back to the starting position.

Things to look for:

- Do you set both hands to the floor at the same time, or do you set one hand down first?

- Can you make the movement as smooth and coordinated as possible?
- When you push yourself away from the floor, does your body stay connected, as though it were one unit, or does one area sag or lift?

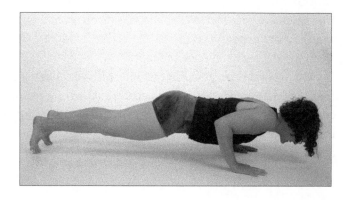

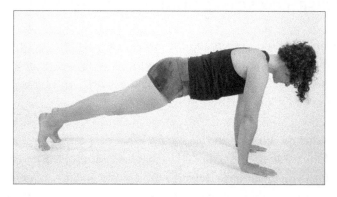

Squat Examples

We have already considered the example of getting up from a chair several times in this book. Let's further explore the act of getting up and down.

EXERCISE: BASIC BOX SQUATS

Begin seated on a chair or box. Hold a medium weight between your hands. Stand up and then sit back down. Repeat this eight to ten times.
   Things to look for:

- Where do your eyes look? Try looking down, straight ahead, and up. Which orientation feels most coordinated?
- Does one hip touch the box sooner than the other? What happens if you focus on both hips touching the box at the same time? How does that feel?
- How wide are your feet? What happens if you place them further apart? What happens if you place them closer together? How does changing the feet influence the motion?
- Do you maintain contact with the floor with your heels and forefoot? Both are important. If the heels are lifting, try maintaining contact between the floor and the center of the heel throughout the movement. If the forefoot is lifting, try maintaining weight across the ball of the foot throughout the movement.

EXERCISE: BOX SQUAT SINGLE-LEG VARIATION

Come into a seated position on the box. Place your left foot on top of your right foot. Keep this foot configuration as you stand up and sit back down. Repeat three to five times and switch sides.

Things to look for:

- What do you do with your hands? What happens if you reach them forward as you stand up? Does that help with control and balance?
- Can you lower back down to the box slowly? If you feel like you are rushing through the movement, see where you can slow down.
- Is one side easier than the other?

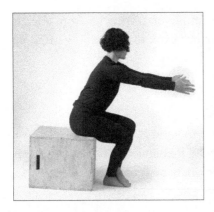 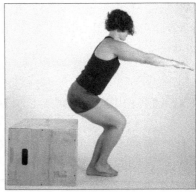

EXERCISE: SPLIT-STANCE GET UP

Imagine you are facing a low table. Reach your arms out in front of you, as though you were setting your hands on the table and shift them slightly to the left so they are oriented over your left leg. Step your right foot back and lower your right knee to the floor.

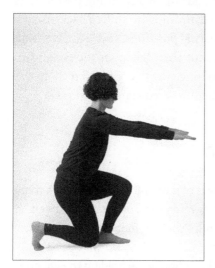 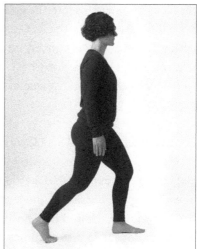

Imagine your hands are pressing down into the table as you press your left foot into the floor and right ball of the foot into the floor to stand up. Repeat three to five times, returning to the starting position each time, and switch sides.

- This movement can be performed holding weights once you are comfortable with the movement in the legs.

Things to look for:

- Does the front heel lift? What happens if you keep it down? Does that change things?
- Are you able to keep the hands oriented over the front leg? Another way to think of this is as though the chest were rotated slightly over the front leg.

- Does your torso stay rigid and upright? What happens if you let your torso hinge forward slightly? Does that change things?
- Is one side more difficult than the other?

Deadlift Examples

Deadlifting starts with a hinge and ends up in a standing position. As the weight comes closer to the ground, the hips are shifted back, usually behind the heels, with the feet in varying positions. If you are working with someone who is concerned about their back, set the weight up relatively high so they don't have to hinge over very far to pick up the weight; you could also use one of the staggered stance versions.

EXERCISE: SUITCASE LOWER

Hold on to two dumbbells or kettlebells of moderate weight. Reach them down along the outside of the legs towards the outside of the heels so the hips move back and the legs bend. Push the feet into the floor and stand up. Repeat four to six times.

Once you get comfortable with the action while holding the weights, you can set the weights on the floor or an elevated surface on the outside of the feet. Pick up the weights and then set them down. Repeat four to six times.

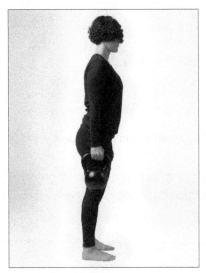 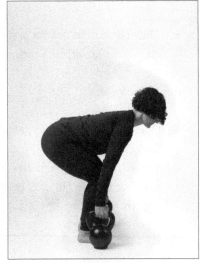

Things to look for:

- It isn't necessary to reach the weights all of the way to the floor. In fact, when you are first learning this exercise, stop before you get to the floor or set up higher targets, like stacked yoga blocks or steps, to aim for.
- Keep the weights touching the outside of the legs as you reach down.
- Can you keep the heels on the ground? If so, can you feel how the heels push into the floor to bring you back up into a standing position?
- Can you hold the weights with a relatively strong grip? Imagine that all five fingers are equally grasping the weight. Does that change your experience at all?

EXERCISE: KICKSTAND DEADLIFT, BACK HEEL ANCHORED, TWO ARM

Hold two moderately heavy weights. Stand so a wall is behind you. Prop your left heel against the wall. The ball of your left foot will be pressing into the ground.

Reach the weights down so they frame your right foot. They don't need to touch the ground, or you can raise the surface by using yoga blocks, steps, or books.

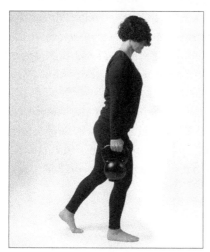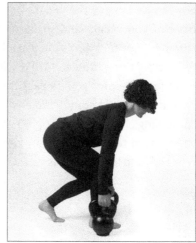

As you reach the weights around your front foot, the butt cheeks reach back, as though they were going to touch the wall. Press through the feet to stand back up. Repeat three to five times and switch sides.

Once you get comfortable with the movement, try beginning with the weights framing the front foot on the floor. Pick the weights up and then set them down. Repeat three to five times and switch sides.

You can also try this with your back heel off the wall. How does that change things for you?

Things to look for:

- Where do your eyes look as you perform the movement? See if you can find a spot in front of you to look at softly while you are lowering the weight around the front foot and lifting it back up.
- Does your front knee bend as you do this movement? Allow the front knee to bend. How does that change things?
- If you are struggling to reach your hips back evenly, try the movement a few times without the weights. Make sure your chest is rotated slightly so it's over the front leg as you do the movement.
- Are you able to press the balls of the back foot and the front foot into the ground to come back up?
- Are you holding the weights with a strong, even grip?

EXERCISE: BETWEEN THE LEGS DEADLIFT

Begin by holding a moderate weight between your hands. Allow your arms to be long so the weight hangs down. Slide the weight down the front of your thighs and shins towards the top of the shoelaces. Press through your feet and slide it back up to the starting position. Repeat four to six times. You can try it with and without the knees bent—see what feels best for you. Repeat three to five times.

Once you are comfortable with the movement, set the weight on something elevated that is right between your feet. Slide the hands down the front of the legs until they can grasp the weight. Press through the feet and hold the weight as you stand back up. Repeat three to five times.

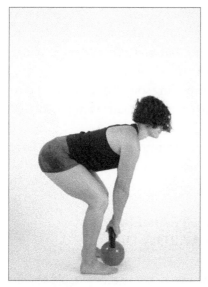 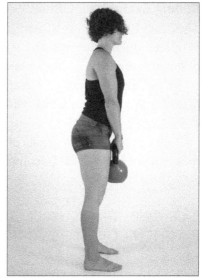

Things to look for:

- Are you able to feel your hips and pelvis reaching back as you slide the weight down the front of the thighs?
- Where do your eyes look? As you come up, imagine that your eyes are reaching in front of you.
- Are you gripping the weight evenly with both hands?
- Did you set the weight up high enough so that it doesn't feel like you are restricted by your flexibility when you pick it up?

There are so many more variations, including single leg, load in single arm, wide stance/sumo deadlift, and straight front-leg staggered stance. If you can get a good sense of how the movement is initiated (from the hips), and how to execute the movement in a way that feels safe and strong, you can access a sense of resiliency throughout the legs and torso.

Pulling Examples

The deadlifting variations above are examples of pulling with the legs. Now let's look at pulling with the arms. But first, what does the image of pulling conjure up? Take a moment and think about it.

When I think of pulling, I imagine pulling something into my body. So, if I am pulling something with my arms, it means I am pulling the object closer to me.

This can happen in a variety of ways. Here are a few exercises I have found that work well for teaching someone the action of pulling.

EXERCISE: RING/SUSPENSION TRAINER/ KITCHEN COUNTER/STAIRWAY ROW UP

Hold on to a suspension trainer, doorway, or some other stable object. You will see me holding on to a pole in the photo below. Walk your feet back a little if necessary so that when you lean back, your arms are straight and your body is at a comfortable angle. Turn your palms so they face each other. Pull yourself up to the rings by letting your elbows bend. Slowly straighten your arms and lower yourself away from the rings. Perform this four to six times, emphasizing the sense of control as you lower down.

You can also do this with just one arm, either allowing the torso to rotate away from the object as you straighten your arm or keeping the torso square to the object the entire time.

Things to look for:

- Does your body move as a unit when you pull up, or does your back arch? Try letting your back arch and then try keeping your body straight, like a plank. Which feels more supported?
- Can you hold the rings or other stable object with an even grip? See if you can feel support from the pinkie side of the hand to the thumb side of the hand.
- Do the insides of your feet lift? What happens if you keep them down? Does that change things for you?
- Are you breathing?
- Do your elbows stay close to your body, or do they rotate outwards? What happens if you keep them close to your body?

- Do your ribs flare forward? What happens if you keep them in?

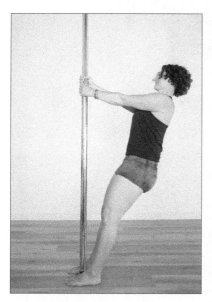 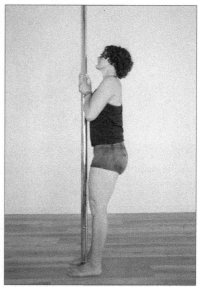

This movement can be done with a variety of hand positions at a variety of different angles, all of which will change the loading patterns on the upper body tissues. Remember that this is a pulling action, so focus on the support coming from the mid-back.

EXERCISE: QUADRUPED ROW

Come into a quadruped position with your hands on two light to medium dumbbells. Press your knees and your left hand into the ground as you row the right elbow back, pulling the dumbbell in your right hand by the right side of your body. Slowly lower it down. Switch sides. Perform six to eight per side.

Things to look for:

- Does your spine shift? If so, can you keep your spine still?
- Does your elbow stay by the side of your body? Can you keep your elbow by the side of your body?
- Can you keep your ribs parallel with the floor?

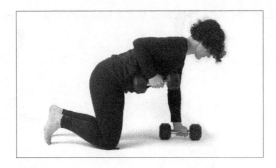

This can be progressed to doing just one side at a time, or you can extend one leg out as you row the opposite arm.

EXERCISE: SEATED BANDED ROW

Come into a seated position with one leg extended and the other knee bent. If this is uncomfortable, you can also do this seated on a chair or with your hips propped up on a blanket. Place the resistance band around the ball of the extended foot, holding both ends of the band in the opposite hand. Pull the band towards the side of your body by bending the elbow. Slowly straighten the arm. Repeat six to eight times.

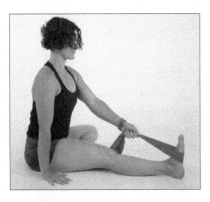 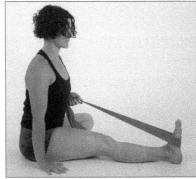

Things to look for:

- Does your torso stay stable as you row, or does it rock forward and back? Can you keep it still as you pull the band?
- When the band is by the side of your body, can you feel your

shoulders moving back? And when the arms are straight, can you feel how the shoulders move forward?

- Are your knees bent? Try bending your knees. See if that feels more stable.

This movement can be done with the band at various levels (chest level, low, high). It can also be done with one arm instead of two or by alternating the movement. Make sure you use a resistance band that is taut enough that is feels like you are challenging the muscles.

In this chapter, I purposefully chose movements that weren't terribly complex and didn't require a lot of equipment. The beauty of strength training is it doesn't have to be complicated to be effective. In fact, I find myself gravitating towards the most basic movements for my own strength-training routine and saving the more complex movements for skill work. Find what works for you and remember that when it comes to building strength, consistency is key.

References

Adhikari R.K., Yadav S.K., & Karn A. (2017). A comparative study of carrying angle with respect to sex and dominant arm in eastern population of Nepal. International Journal of Current Research and Review, 9(7), 19-22.

Andersen V., Fimland M.S., Mo D.-A., Iversen V.M., et al. (2019). Electromyographic comparison of the barbell deadlift using constant versus variable resistance in healthy, trained men. PLOS ONE, 14(1), 1-12.

Brewer C. (2017). Chapter 10: Developing Functional Strength Progressions, 281-340. In: Athletic Movement Skills: Training for Sports Performance. Champaign, IL: Human Kinetics.

Brun C., Giogi N., Pinard A.-M., Gagne M., McCabe C.S., & Mercier C. (2019). Exploring the relationships between altered body perception, limb position sense, and limb movement sense in complex regional pain syndrome. Journal of Pain, 20(1), 17-27.

Bundy D.T., Szarma N., Pahwa M., & Leuthardt E. (2018). Unilateral, 3D arm movement kinematics are encoded in ipsilateral human cortex. Journal of Neuroscience, 38(47), 10042-10056.

De Almeida T.B.C., Dobashi E.T., Nishimi A.Y., De Almeida Junrion E.B., Pascarelli L., & Rodrigueq L.M.R. (2017). Analysis of the pattern and mechanism of elbow injuries related to armbar-type armlocks in jiu-jitsu fighters. Acta Ortopédica Brasileira, 25(5), 209-211.

Elias A.R.C., Hammill C.D., & Mizner R.L. (2015). Changes in quadriceps and hamstring cocontraction following landing instruction in patients with anterior cruciate ligament reconstruction. Journal of Orthopaedic & Sports Physical Therapy, 45(4), 273-280.

Gong X., Chen Y., Chang J., Huang Y., Cai M., & Zhang M. (2018). Environmental enrichment reduces adolescent anxiety- and depression-like behaviors of rats subjected to infant nerve injury. Journal of Neuroinflammation, 15, 262.

Heitmann S., Ferris N., & Breakspear M. (2012). Muscle co-contraction modulates damping and joint stability in a three-link biomechanical limb. Frontiers in Neurorobotics, 5, 5.

Herzog W., Powers K., Johnston K., & Duvall M. (2015). A new paradigm for muscle contraction. Frontiers in Physiology, 6, 174.

Hirji Z., Hunan J.S., & Choudur H.N. (2011). Imaging of the bursae. Journal of Clinical Imaging Science, 1(1), 1-9.

Ito J., & Tsuji T. (1992). Redundant degrees of freedom and motor impedance control in human movements. Biomechanisms, 11, 223-233.

Jackson P., & Neumann D.A. (2019). Chapter 3: Structure and Function of Skeletal Muscle, 34-49. Essentials of Kinesiology for the Physical Therapist Assistant. Cambridge, MA: Elsevier.

Kim D., & Hwang J.M. (2018). The center of pressure and ankle muscle co-contraction in response to anterior-posterior perturbations. PLOS ONE, 13(11), e0207667.

Kubo K., Kanehisa H., & Fukunaga T. (2001). Effects of different duration isometric contractions on tendon elasticity in human quadriceps muscles. Journal of Physiology, 536(Pt 2), 649-655.

Latash M.L., Levin M.F., Scholz J.P., & Schoner G. (2010). Motor control theories and their applications. Medicina (Kaunas), 46(6), 382-392.

Lee D.-K., Kang M.-H., Jang J.-H., An D.-H., Yoo W.-G., & Oh J.-S. (2012). Effects of changing the resistance direction using an elastic tubing band on abdominal muscle activities during isometric upper limb exercises. Journal of Physical Therapy Science, 24(8), 703-706.

Linaker C.H., & Walker-Bone K. (2015). Shoulder disorders and occupation. Best Practice Researchers in Clinical Rheumatology, 29(3), 405-423.

Lipman K., Wang C., Ting K., Soo C., & Zheng Z. (2018). Tendinopathy: Injury, repair, and current exploration. Drug Design, Development and Therapy, 12, 591-603.

Lombardi J.A., Surburg P., Eklund S., & Koceja D. (2000). Age differences and changes in midline-crossing inhibition in the lower extremities. Journals of Gerontology Series A, 55(5), 293-298.

Ludewig P.M., & Reynolds J.F. (2009). The association of scapular kinematics and glenohumeral joint pathologies. Journal of Orthopedic Sports and Physical Therapy, 39(2), 90-104.

Lustenberger D.P., Ng V.Y., Best T.M., & Ellis T.J. (2011). Efficacy of treatment of trochanteric bursitis: A systematic review. Clinical Journal of Sports Medicine, 21(5), 447-453.

Mulder T. (2007). Motor imagery and action observation: Cognitive tools for rehabilitation. Journal of Neural Transmission, 114(10), 1265-1278.

Nakamura Y., Uchiyama S., Kamimura M., Komatsu M., Ikegami S., & Kato H. (2016). Bone alterations are associated with ankle osteoarthritis joint pain. Scientific Reports, 6, 18717.

Nunes M., Martins e Silva D., Moreira R., et al. (2016). Motor irradiation according to the concept of proprioceptive neuromuscular facilitation: Measurement tools and future prospects. International Journal of Physical Medicine & Rehabilitation, 4(2), 1000330.

Osawa Y., Studenski S.A., & Ferrucci L. (2018). Knee extension rate of torque development and peak torque: Associations with lower extremity function. Journal of Cachexia Sarcopenia Muscle, 9(3), 530-539.

Pakenham D.O., Quinn A.J., Fry A., Francis S.T., et al. (2020). Post-stimulus beta responses are modulated by task duration. Neuroimage, 206, 116288.

Prinold J.A.I., & Bull A.M.J. (2016). Scapula kinematics of pull-up techniques: Avoiding impingement risk with training changes. Journal of Science and Medicine in Sport, 19(8), 629-635.

Reid D. (2016). The management of greater trochanteric pain syndrome: A literature review. Journal of Orthopedics, 13(1), 15-28.

Shemmell J., Krutky M.A., & Perrault E.J. (2010). Stretch sensitive reflexes as an adaptive mechanism for maintaining limb stability. Clinical Neurophysiology, 121(10), 1680-1689.

Sood A., Paik A., & Lee E. (2013). Dupuytren's contracture. Eplasty, 13, ic1.

Speers C.J.B., & Bhogal G.S. (2017). Greater trochanteric pain syndrome: A review of diagnosis and management in general practice. British Journal of General Practice, 67(663), 479-480.

Summers J.J., Kagerer F.A., Garry M.I., Hiraga C.Y., Loftus A., & Cauraugh J.H. (2007). Bilateral and unilateral movement training on upper limb function in chronic stroke patients: A TMS study. Journal of the Neurological Sciences, 252(1), 76-82.

Whitall J., Waller S.M., Sorkin J.D., Forrester L.W., et al. (2011). Bilateral and unilateral arm training in motor function through differing neuroplastic mechanisms: A single-blinded randomized controlled trial. Neurorehabilitation and Neural Repair, 25(2), 118-129.

CHAPTER 8

Mobility: Practical Application

I have a client who isn't naturally very flexible. His spine, shoulders, and hips all have a tendency to feel stiff. As a result, he starts his morning by stretching and doing targeted mobility work. It makes his body feel better and puts him in a better mood. When he comes to see me, particularly on days after he has played golf, we spend extra time moving different areas in a thoughtful, directed way. He becomes more animated as the session goes on and his body becomes more flexible. I don't think that's coincidental.

Not everyone struggles with building strength. There are people for whom strength training is a regular part of their lives, yet they still experience anxiety and a lack of comfort in their physical bodies.

In psychology, specific muscular holding patterns that cause tension or decrease ease in movement are sometimes referred to as body armoring (Greene & Goodrich-Dunn, 2004). Armoring can reduce range of motion throughout the physical structure and happens for a variety of reasons. If the only way someone feels in control is by moving in a very specific manner without much variety, or the person feels a perpetual sense something bad is about to happen, their movement reflects this by becoming less fluid and more rigid.

Language can also influence how someone holds themselves and their beliefs about what types of movements should be avoided because they are potentially harmful. Remember how in Chapters 4 and 6 we talked about the importance of active listening for effective coaching? The art of communication can directly impact whether someone follows through on a suggested home exercise program or takes your suggestion to prioritize sleep rather than staying up late surfing the internet.

How you talk about movement can either empower your client to try new things, or prompt them to avoid certain exercises or movements because they are worried about doing it wrong or injuring themselves (Main *et al.*, 2010). If, for instance, you are working with someone who was told by a professional that flexing the spine is bad and causes disc damage because discs are like jelly donuts, chances are high your client will avoid flexing the spine at all costs and will reach towards the floor in an interesting, guarded way.

Confession: I struggled with armoring for a combination of the reasons above until I turned 30. This is a topic I understand and relate to fully, and it's important, just like understanding hypermobility is important. If someone is stiff for reasons rooted in more than just muscular tightness, as you help them unravel their ability to move more freely and instill in them a sense of physical freedom they may never have experienced, it wouldn't be unusual for them to experience initial mental resistance followed by motor control confusion. I will discuss this more in Chapter 9, but first, let's look at neurological tightness versus muscular stiffness.

Neurological Tightness versus Muscular Stiffness

In Chapter 4, I discussed how mechanoreceptors send sensory information about the body to the CNS. Inside skeletal muscle fibers there are fluid-filled capsules made up of connective tissue. These capsules contain intrafusal fibers, which are specialized muscle fibers responsible for providing afferent information to the CNS (Colon *et al.*, 2017).

This structure is called a muscle spindle and is innervated by specialized nerve cells that detect changes in muscle length. When a muscle is stretched, the nerve cell fires rapidly; when the stretch decreases, the nerve cell fires less rapidly.

This finely tuned response to changes in muscle length allows the CNS to detect both small and large changes in the length of the muscle. These specialized nerve cells are also sensitive to how fast and in which direction the muscle is changing length. The CNS regulates the loading of the muscle; there are specialized neurons that modulate muscle-spindle activity. These neurons allow the muscle to transition from stretch to contraction smoothly (Cuoco & Tyler, 2012).

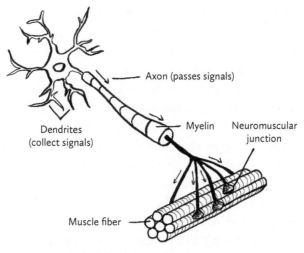

Axon (passes signals)

Dendrites
(collect signals)

Myelin

Neuromuscular
junction

Muscle fiber

NEUROMUSCULAR JUNCTION

You are probably beginning to notice that the CNS (brain and spinal cord) is getting constant feedback from the PNS (nerves in the body, organs, and everything else). When people begin to feel the connection between what they experience physically and what they are feeling emotionally, it creates an opportunity to feel different by moving differently.

The muscle spindle isn't the only mechanoreceptor sensitive to the detection of muscle length. Golgi tendon organs (GTOs), which are usually located at the place where muscle becomes tendon (or tendon becomes muscle), aka the myotendinous junction, are collagenous bundles supplied by lots of sensory nerves. When these bundles stretch, they become straighter. This causes the nerve fibers to fire more rapidly. They, too, are sensitive to small changes in muscle tension, and while most of the stretch is absorbed by muscle spindles, GTOs are more sensitive to detecting active muscle contraction that stresses the myotendinous junction (Smith & Plowman, 2006).

It's important to note that the myotendinous junction is the primary site of force transmission. When you move and force is being transmitted from the foot to the tibia to the femur, the myotendinous junction is what allows that transmission. The GTOs are an important part of sensing that force detection. If someone has a more sensitive nervous system and feels pain during certain movements, making a small change in foot position or how the shin moves forward will often change the way they experience the movement.

If someone is struggling with feeling pain in their shoulders during a push-up and I change the movement so that instead of doing a push-up, they shift back to down dog, lower down onto their stomach, and then push themselves back up into a straight-arm plank position before shifting back to down dog again, the different loading patterns in the upper body may totally change the sensation of pain in their shoulders. Or if I have them turn their fingers out, or place more weight on the pinkie side of the hand, or stagger the hand position, it may also change their experience of discomfort. Changing the load by changing position or coordination changes the experience.

Researchers have suggested that how frequently the muscle spindles fire during muscle stretch isn't only related to muscle length and velocity. A number of things in a person's history can impact their ability to detect and respond to muscle stretch and they can be fleeting. For instance, if you do a hamstring stretch that is held for a specific amount of time, the firing rate of the muscle spindle decreases (Blum *et al.*, 2017). This is not a permanent change; if you perform a relaxed, static hamstring stretch on Monday during your workout to try and decrease the sensation of tightness in your hamstrings, when you wake up on Tuesday and do the same stretch, your hamstrings will probably feel tight even if they felt looser when you finished your stretch on Monday. If, however, you apply the same intervention three times a week for six weeks, you will notice your range of motion in that specific intervention improving. The logical conclusion would be that the muscle is becoming physically less tight, enabling you to access the position more easily. Muscle is made up of material that changes shape in response to the force applied to it; when clients feel the sensation of stretch, the image many have in their heads is of the muscle pulling like taffy, as though the muscle were getting longer. The thing is, though, that muscle is three-dimensional, just like our physical shape is three-dimensional and dependent on more than just the muscle itself. The ability of a muscle to physically get longer is determined by not only the muscle's extensibility (defined as a muscle's ability to extend to a predetermined end point), but by capsular structures as well (Weppler & Magnusson, 2010).

Research (*ibid.*) has suggested that muscles are viscoelastic, which means that if a force is applied that causes the muscle to change shape, the muscle returns to its original shape once the force is removed. Muscles are considered viscous because of the way they respond to tensile force—they are rate and time dependent. This means the longer you pull on them and how often you pull on them causes slow changes in length. Imagine that your hamstring muscle is like syrup in the bottom of the container—you have to hold the container tipped for a while in order for the syrup to actually come out, and when it does finally begin to exit, it does so slowly and only if the container is tipped the entire time.

This viscoelastic nature of muscles means that there is always passive muscle tension occurring that prevents the muscle from stretching too far. You can never really get all of the syrup out of the container because of this tension. The passive tension is the result of structural properties of the muscle and surrounding fascia; active tension is provided by reflexive contraction—basically, your CNS gets a little nervous when you push your muscle into a new position and says, "Hmm. I don't know that this is a good idea, so I am going to put on the brakes" (Page, 2012). This is different than the syrup, which doesn't have a CNS to step in, so it continues to ooze slowly out of the container with no real stopping point.

If you come into a wide-legged forward fold position and set a timer for three minutes, there is a high probability you will be folded further forward at the end of the three minutes (this isn't true 100 percent of the time—we will talk about exceptions a little later in the chapter). What accounts for the improvement in flexibility?

One potential cause of increased flexibility is sensory tolerance, or an increased willingness to tolerate the discomfort initially associated with the stretch. This may happen because of psychological beliefs: "If I stretch, I will become more flexible. Since I am stretching, I am becoming more flexible." What is actually happening is the person's perception that stretching will make them more flexible is altering their experience of the sensation.

Increased flexibility may also happen because the person becomes more tolerant of the stretch sensation so it becomes quieter; the loudness is dampened by repeated exposure and a realization by the entire system that the range of motion the body is being exposed to isn't harmful and can be tolerated for longer periods of time (Law et al., 2009).

If you asked two people of roughly the same fitness levels—one of whom has a naturally high degree of flexibility while the other can't touch their toes—to perform the same stretch, would their experiences be the same?

"Of course not, Jenn. They are two different people. Their experiences would be different because they have different histories and perspectives." Valid point. What I should have asked was would their experience of stretch sensation be the same?

No. There is a strong chance the person with natural flexibility would think stretching felt "good," while the naturally stiff person would make a face and say they felt tight or that stretching felt uncomfortable. One possible explanation for their different experiences of the position is that they have different tolerances.

Does flexibility even really matter? Yes, because it gives us options. Chapter 7 showed that variation is beneficial for motor control, movement efficiency, and loading throughout the musculoskeletal system. When you have adequate joint mobility, you have more options, which in beneficial for not only movement but also mental well-being. When you can move in a lot of different ways throughout your environment without fear of injury, you begin to experience more security and freedom in how you move. This trickles over into other areas of your life. Physically flexibility influences mental flexibility.

Of course, this begs the question: how much flexibility does an individual need? It depends on the person's goals. Let's say Jack, a 55-year-old runner, finds it difficult to bend over to put on his shoes while standing. He wants to be able to make it through his life without throwing his back out, and he wants to keep running. Gaining enough mobility to get up and down off the floor comfortably in a variety of ways and being able to tie his shoes without feeling like he might potentially break would be adequate starting places for improving Jack's flexibility.

In contrast, Jessica, a 42-year-old fitness enthusiast, wants to be able to press to handstand but has trouble bending forward in a wide straddle position. She can comfortably sit in a low squat and is regularly complimented on her shoulder flexibility. She needs to work on end-range strength and flexibility in the wide straddle position, something Jack currently doesn't need or want. She will use more targeted flexibility and strength work to improve her motor control, strength, and flexibility in the wide straddle position. She needs different flexibility than Jack to accomplish her goals, though, unlike Jack, she currently has enough flexibility to feel comfortable moving throughout her everyday life.

There are many neurological tricks in the mobility world that lead to short-term results. All of them involve integrating more senses (e.g., touch, vision, smell, proprioception). Sensorimotor integration is an individual's ability to incorporate sensory inputs about the external environment and use that information to inform and shape subsequent movement (Edwards *et al.*, 2019). When an individual is able to incorporate multiple senses, the brain has a more complete picture about the most effective and efficient way to move. Anecdotally, this appears to downregulate the nervous system and make movement output less guarded or rigid, possibly because the nervous system has more information to work with—information leads to more informed movement decisions.

What ideas can you begin to formulate about mobility for the stiff, perfectionistic client who has a baseline of strength and endurance?

There is no right answer here, and there different ways this could be approached. I am going to outline the approach that I have found useful for slowly chipping away at the guarding that some of us use to deal with the stresses of everyday life. As the nervous system shifts and the muscles become less taut, the musculoskeletal system also begins to deal with load differently. Fortunately, this usually leads to more efficient load tolerance, but that doesn't mean there's no initial adjustment period. When I first began introducing more hip-mobility work into my practice, I got occasional nerve twinges in my knees during my morning runs for about three weeks. I wasn't concerned because I could feel I was changing, and sure enough, the twinges gradually lessened during the course of the three weeks until they disappeared completely.

I have witnessed similar things with other clients who are wired like me—there is a brief adjustment period and then the shifting becomes a new normal. (Similar things happen when people first begin building strength; they are asking their entire system to adjust to a new way of being. I mention this because there is often fear around these sensations, but as long as they disappear and don't last, they aren't anything to be concerned about. Some people are more susceptible to sensations during this rewiring period than others.)

Approaching Mobility

In the context of this book, think of mobility as exposure to new positions. These new positions can be done at a single joint or throughout multiple joints. You can introduce positions that improve mobility in the hands, feet, back, hips, shoulders, or throughout the entire structure. When you are first introducing mobility to someone, what do you think feels more safe—working on flexibility in multiple or individual joints?

Usually, it feels safer to work on individual joints, but this is not always the case. There are certain positions which require several joints to integrate together that can be both downregulating and effective. I usually use a combination of addressing isolated joints and integration.

Generally, one of the easiest ways to set people up for mobility success and not overwhelm their systems is to teach it the same way you would strength. If you use thoughtful progressions, listen to your client's feedback, and expose them repeatedly over a period of time to similar mobility patterns, their coordination and tolerance to the positions will improve.

Mobility work also taps into the concepts we discussed around mindful movement in Chapter 5. Because mobility work tends to require a bit of focused attention, whether you are using external tasks to work on movement variability or more internally based instructions, following the foundations of mindful movement ensures a sense of internal strength and connection. Do you remember what those foundations are?

Breathing, grounding, centering, and listening are the fundamental building blocks of mindful movement. In a mobility context, breathing can be used to monitor stress; it can also be used to create an internal sense of stability or to mobilize the thoracic spine. See Chapter 5 if you need a recap.

Mobility Sequences

When I am first working with someone who has a lot of stiffness, I generally begin by helping them feel their spine, hands, and feet. When the spine is able to move and respond to perturbations, it becomes easier for them to feel where their center is. When the hands, feet, and ankles are able to allow movement and provide strength, they can respond to the floor, supporting the physical structure and creating a sense of grounding.

It's important to remember that subtle movements are enough to send sensory feedback information to the CNS. When you are working with someone who is stiff and fearful that mobility work may be injurious, using subtle movements (especially in the spine and pelvis) will actually decrease SNS activity and open a window for more movement—basically, the stiff person will become more flexible by being able to feel small changes in position.

Mobility work can be implemented throughout a session, as a rest between strength work, or it can be a standalone modality. Mobility work and strength work are two sides of the same coin, complementing each other and creating opportunities for more variation and a greater sense of physical control.

As you explore the mobility sequences outlined throughout the rest of this chapter, remember that these are only ideas and this is in no way an exhaustive list of mobility possibilities. When people present with a lot of stiffness, I generally use gentle mobility work in the beginning; as they grow more confident and their holding patterns shift because they are moving more easily, I move into more active work. (The reverse is true when someone has a high degree of mobility—I use more active work initially to ensure a greater sense of stability.)

Mobility Sequence I: Emphasis on Spine, Ankles, and Wrists

SEATED HEAD NODS

Begin in a seated position. Nod the chin up. Nod the chin down.

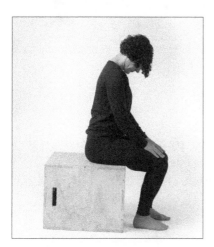 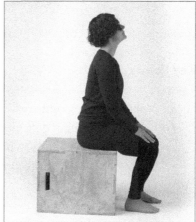

Key Points

- Try leading with the eyes. Try keeping the eyes still. Try it without thinking about the eyes. Which feels more natural?

- Play with altering the head position at slightly different angles to change the experience.

SEATED RIB NODS

In a seated position, move your ribs up, flaring your chest. Move your ribs down, collapsing your chest. Go back and forth between the two positions. Which position feels more natural?

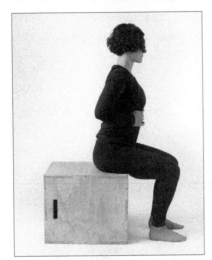 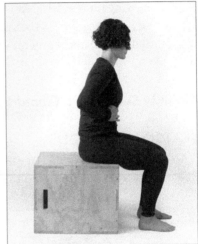

Key Points

- Make the movement small.
- If you are having a difficult time, try placing your hands on your ribs and use the hands to help guide the movement.
- Play with altering the position of the torso to change the experience.

SEATED BELLY BUTTON MOVEMENT

In a seated position, move your belly button forward. Move your belly button backward. Which part of your spine is moving?
Does this feel easier or harder than the head and ribs?

Perform each movement six to eight times with an emphasis on feeling the feet against the floor and noticing how the pelvis changes position in each position.

Key Points

- Make the movement small.
- Reflect on which areas are easier and which are more difficult.
- Check in with the breath occasionally. Is there tension in the jaw? Are you breathing?

SEATED-POSITION WRIST FLEXION AND EXTENSION WITH FISTS AND WITH OPEN HANDS

From a seated position, reach your arms straight out in front of you with your palms facing towards the ceiling. Extend the wrist, flexing the fingers towards the floor. Return the hand to the starting position.

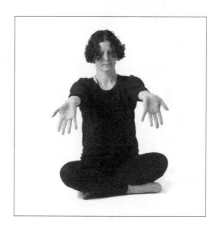

Perform six to eight repetitions. Vary the hand position slightly for a different experience.

Key Points

- Make the movement small.
- Keep the arms straight and isolate the movement at the wrists.
- Maintain contact with the floor. If you are seated on the floor, be sure to feel a connection with the ischial tuberosities (sitting bones). If you are seated in a chair, feel the sitting bones and the feet against the floor.
- Check in with the jaw. Is it tense? Are you able to breathe easily?
- Is there tension in the shoulders?
- Are you keeping the rest of yourself relatively still?

CLOSED-CHAIN WRIST EXTENSION IN THREE DIFFERENT POSITIONS AGAINST A WALL OR BENCH

The wrists can feel sensitive, so remember to work slowly and use a position you can comfortably tolerate. Place your fingertips against a wall or bench. Slowly allow the palm to come towards the wall/bench. Hold in the fully extended position, actively reaching the heel of the palm towards the wall for two or three breaths. Relax, and change the orientation of the hands.

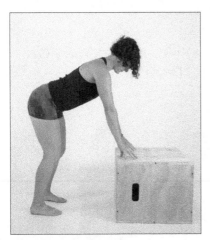 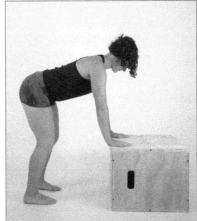

Key Points

- Keep the torso relatively still.
- Keep the elbows relatively straight.
- Remember to breathe.
- For an added bonus, when the wrists are in the fully extended position, remove the left hand from the bench and trace the outline of the right hand with the left index finger. Place the left hand on the bench and do the same thing with the right hand. Pause for a moment with both hands on the bench. Do they feel different?

ANKLE AND FOOT AWARENESS, SUPINE

Lie down on your back with your knees bent and your feet flat. Feel the feet connecting to the floor.

Lift the front of the right foot off the floor (the back of the right heel will still be in contact with the floor). Reach the right heel away from you, allowing the leg to extend.

Once the leg is extended, keep it there. Pull the right heel towards you (the toes will point away from you). Reach the right heel away from you. Repeat this six to eight times, pulling the heel towards you and reaching it away from you with the leg extended.

Once you have finished, pull the right heel towards you, allowing the right knee to bend until the foot is flat on the floor. Take a moment to observe the foot against the floor and then switch sides, performing the same action with the left foot.

Key Points

- Are the fingers quiet, or are they moving as the ankle moves?
- Is one side easier than the other?
- Can you feel where the center of the heels are in relation to the rest of the foot?

STANDING ANKLE MOBILITY, EMPHASIS ON THE FOREFOOT

Stand facing a wall with your fingertips lightly on the wall. Imagine that there is a line connecting the center of your head to the ceiling. Lift your heels away from the floor. Don't let the center of your head move off center. (Another way to think of this is that the head and torso are moving as a unit, so the back doesn't bend or extend.)

As you lift, see if you can feel the weight evenly across the balls of your feet. You can play with the weight distribution while your heels are away from the floor, rocking the weight to the pinkie-toe side of the foot and the big-toe side of the foot until you have a good sense of even weight distribution.

Slowly lower your heels to the floor, feeling the heels as they connect with the ground. Repeat this movement six to eight times.

Key Points

- Are you able to move your body and head together by lifting the heels?
- When you consciously keep the weight even across the feet, does that feel comfortable or unusual?
- Can you feel both heels when they return to the floor?
- Are you remembering to breathe?

SPINAL MOBILITY, INTEGRATION

Come onto a forearms and knees position so your elbows are under your shoulders and your knees are under your hips. Shift your hips back towards your heels. Shift your hips to the starting position over your knees.

Go back and forth, shifting the hips towards the heels and over the knees four to six times, allowing the spine to respond to the movement. After your last one, perform four more repetitions without allowing the spine to respond to the movement. How does that feel? Is it different?

Key Points

- Do your hips move back evenly or do they veer towards one side?
- Can you maintain the connection of your forearms against the floor when you shift your hips back?
- Do you prefer the top of the feet against the floor, or do you prefer your toes flexed back towards you?
- Are you breathing?

Before moving on, take a moment to think about how you could slightly alter each of the exercises in this sequence. Write down one or two ideas for each. Here are a couple of quick ideas:

- Seated Head Nods, Seated Rib Nods and Seated Belly Button Movement: Stagger the elbows on the knees.
- Seated-Position Wrist Flexion and Extension with Fists and with Open Hands: Alternate the hands.
- Closed-Chain Wrist Flexion in Three Different Positions against a Wall or Bench: Place one hand higher than the other on the wall or ahead of the other on the bench.
- Ankle and Foot Awareness, Supine: Don't extend the leg all of the way out or allow the foot to turn out (or in).
- Standing Ankle Mobility, Emphasis on the Forefoot: Turn the heels away from each other while performing the movement.
- Spinal Mobility, Integration: Stagger the arms or knees.

The beauty of introducing variety is there is no right or wrong answer. I have no doubt your list is different than mine, and that's fantastic. The more you learn to think creatively, the easier it will be to come up with solutions if you introduce a movement that doesn't work for someone. Sometimes the right answer is to abandon the exercise altogether, but often, a slight alteration in position can dramatically improve a person's experience.

Mobility Sequence II: Emphasis on Pelvis, Shoulders, Hands, and Ankles

SUPINE PELVIC TILTS

Lie on your back, with your knees bent and your feet flat on the floor. Gently press the small of your back towards the floor. Gently roll the small of your back away from the floor. Go back and forth between these two positions four to six times.

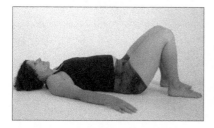
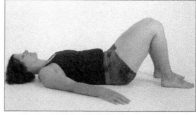

Key Points

- Can you isolate the initiation of the movement to the pelvis, or are other parts of the spine initiating the movement? What happens if you initiate the movement with the pelvis?
- Which parts of your spine respond to the movement? Can you feel echoes of the movement up as high as the head?
- Are you initiating the movement by pushing the feet into the floor? Try it a few times—push the feet into the floor to posteriorly tilt the pelvis and relax the feet to anteriorly tilt the pelvis. Now try the same action without using the feet. Can you feel the difference?
- Are you breathing?
- Are you tensing anywhere in the rest of the body? If you feel like you are tensing or bracing anywhere, can you relax?

TALL KNEELING PELVIC TILTS

Come into a tall kneeling position (it will look like you are standing on your knees). Place your hands so they are resting gently on your thighs. Gently move your pelvis back, away from your hands, and forwards, towards your hands, repeating four to six times.

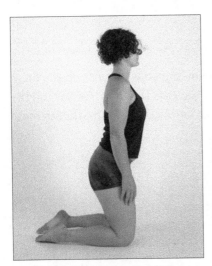 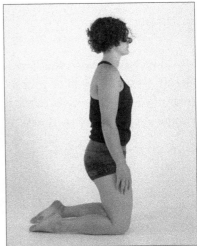

Key Points

- Does it feel like one side moves more easily than the other?
- What happens in your legs when you gently tilt the pelvis forward and back?
- Can you keep your jaw relaxed?
- Are you breathing?

ELBOW ROTATIONS

This can be done: standing, with the hands against a wall; standing, with the hands against an elevated surface, like a chair or bench; on the floor, with the hands on the ground. I am going to describe the version with the hands on the ground, but if you lack wrist extension, please use one of the other variations.

Come into a quadruped position with your wrists under your shoulders and your knees under your hips. Rotate the elbows out. Rotate the elbows in. Go back and forth between these two positions six to eight times. Keep the arms straight as you rotate the elbows.

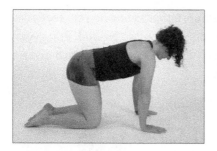 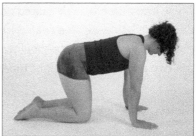

Key Points

- Does your torso stay strong and supportive, or does it collapse while you are rotating the elbows?
- Can you feel how the weight shifts in your hands when you rotate the elbows?
- Is one direction easier than the other?
- Are you remembering to breathe?

STANDING CLOSED-CHAIN HAND AWARENESS

Stand facing a wall. Place your hands on the wall so that the heels of the palms are against the wall (your elbows can be bent if necessary). Lift the thumbs away from the wall three or four times without changing the position of the arms. Now lift the index fingers three or four times, followed by the middle fingers, fourth fingers, and pinkie fingers.

Rest your hands by your sides and observe how they feel.

Key Points

- Are you clenching your jaw?
- Which fingers lift most easily? Which are harder to lift?
- Are you breathing?
- Do your elbows bend when you lift your fingers? Can you prevent them from bending?

OPEN-CHAIN SCAPULAR RETRACTION AND PROTRACTION

Come into a comfortable seated position, either sitting on your feet as in the image below or on a chair with your feet on the ground. Bring your shoulders back. Bring your shoulders forward. Go back and forth between the two positions six to eight times.

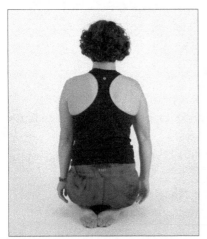 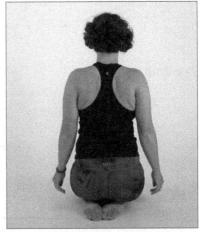

Key Points

- Does your head jut forward when your shoulders move back? Can you perform the movement and keep the head still?
- Can you feel your shoulder blades (scapulae) moving when you bring the shoulders forward and back? Perform a few more, focusing on how the shoulder blades move when you move your shoulders. What direction do the shoulder blades move when your shoulders move forward? What direction do they move when the shoulders move back?
- Are you breathing?

CLOSED-CHAIN SCAPULAR PROTRACTION AND RETRACTION

Come into a quadruped position. The hands can face whichever direction is most comfortable for you. Allow your shoulder blades to move together and apart. If you struggle with this, think about moving the shoulders back and forward, just like you did in the previous exercise. If you are still struggling, allow the chest to move towards the floor and away from the floor. As you do this, see if you can feel the shoulder blades moving. Go back and forth between these two positions six to eight times. On the last one, take two breaths when the shoulder blades are retracted. Move the shoulder blades away from each other and take two breaths, thinking about breathing between the shoulder blades.

Key Points

- Is it easier for you to move the shoulder blades together or apart?
- Can you maintain a firm connection with the elbows and forearms against the wall the entire time? Do a few more, thinking about keeping the elbows and forearms firmly pressing into the wall.
- Is it easier to breathe when the shoulder blades are retracted or protracted?

TALL KNEELING SIT BACKS

Come into a tall kneeling position. Place your feet in whichever position is most comfortable for them. Sit back towards your heels. Don't go so far it feels uncomfortable, just sit back far enough that you feel in control. Return to the starting position. Do this four to six times. Once you have finished, shift the feet so they're in the less comfortable position (so if the top of your foot was flat against the floor, flex the foot so the toes are standing into the floor or vice versa). Try sitting back towards your heels in this position and return to the tall kneeling position. Repeat four to six times.

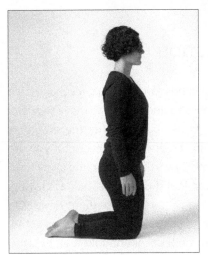 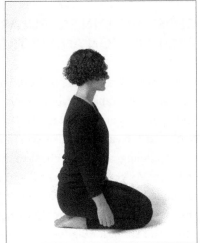

Key Points

- What foot position do you prefer?
- Can you remember not to go to the point of discomfort?
- Does it feel easier as you go along?
- Are you breathing?
- Be aware that someone who is initially extremely tight will unlock more degrees of freedom if they don't go to the point of discomfort.

If there is sensitivity in the low back during pelvic tilts, don't go in the direction that causes sensation. Instead, you can ask the person to imagine what it would be like to move in a pain-free way, without discomfort. It's entirely plausible that after visualizing it a few times, the client will be able to perform the movement in a pain-free way.

It's also possible that the client may not be able to do supine pelvic tilts in a pain-free way but may have no trouble performing tall kneeling or seated pelvic tilts. Even though the supine position should technically feel more safe because of the ground feedback, occasionally people will try to over-recruit their abdominal musculature to perform the movement instead of performing it in a relaxed manner. When this happens, I usually eliminate the supine variation for a couple of weeks while we work on other variations and then return to it once the client understands how to perform the action in a more easeful way.

Spend the next few minutes quickly jotting down ways you could introduce variation to the exercises above. Here is a list of one or two variations per exercise:

- Supine Pelvic Tilts: Lift the front of the feet or lift the heels and perform pelvic tilts.
- Tall Kneeling Pelvic Tilts: Make the legs wide. Make the legs narrow. If in seated, come into long sit or straddle sit.
- Elbow Rotations: Change the direction both fingers are pointing (or change the position of just one hand).
- Standing Closed-Chain Hand Awareness: Take one hand away from the wall, focusing on one hand at a time.
- Open-Chain Scapular Retraction and Protraction: Alternate the shoulders.
- Closed-Chain Scapular Protraction and Retraction: Place one hand higher than the other, or do one arm at a time. Angle the toes out. Angle the toes in.
- Tall Kneeling Sit Backs: Sit over your left heel. Sit over your right heel.

Mobility Sequence III: Spine, Shoulders, and Hips

QUADRUPED SPINAL CIRCLES

Come into a quadruped position or a forearms and knees position. Move your belly button in a circle, bringing it to the right, up, to the left and down. Perform four to six times and then switch directions. Allow your spine to respond to the movement.

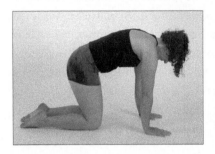 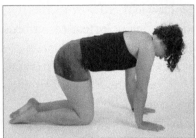

Key Points

- Do your hands and knees stay in contact with the floor while you move your spine in a circular motion?
- Does your head respond to the movement?
- Can you feel the weight transfer across the hands and knees while the spine moves?
- Are you breathing?
- Can you initiate the movement with the breastbone instead of the belly button? Does that feel different? How?

SPLIT-STANCE HIP SHIFT

Come into a tall kneeling position. Take your right foot forward so your right knee is in line with your right hip and your right foot is under your right knee.

Square your hips to the front of the room and make sure your right foot is connected to the floor. Imagine that you have a triangle on the bottom of your right foot that's connecting the center of the right heel, the big-toe ball of the foot, and the pinkie-toe ball of the foot. Keep the triangle firmly pressing down.

Shift your hips forward. Shift your hips back. Go back and forth between these two positions six to eight times.

On your last one, find a place that feels centered and stable. Reach your left arm back like it's going to touch the wall behind you, and then reach it up towards the ceiling, like it's going to touch the ceiling. Go back and forth between these two positions six to eight times. Switch sides and repeat the entire sequence on the other side.

You can also try this movement with the front heel barely lifted from the ground and the weight even across the ball of the foot, from the big toe to the pinkie toe. How does that change things?

Key Points

- As you shift the hips forward, are you arching your back? Can you shift the hips forward without arching your back?
- Are you keeping a connection with the heel of the front foot as you shift forward? If the heel of the front foot lifts, can you find a way to perform the movement without lifting the right heel (maybe make it smaller)?
- What position is your back foot in? What happens if you place it the other way? Is it more or less comfortable?
- Are you breathing?
- When you reach your arms, does your spine shift position? Can you keep your spine still?
- When you reach your hand behind you, does it go straight back or does it move towards the center of the body? Can you reach it straight back?
- Is one side easier than the other?

SHOULDER SHRUGS, TWO WAYS

Come into a tall kneeling position. Shrug your shoulders up by your ears. Shrug your shoulders down. Perform this six to eight times.

Place your forearms on the floor and perform the same movement, shrugging the shoulders up towards your ears and down towards your hips. Perform this six to eight times.

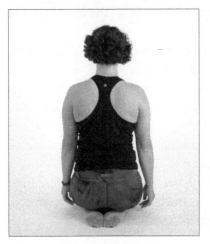 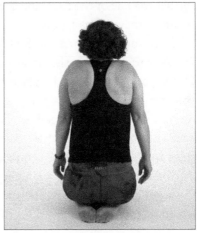

Key Points

- Does your neck move when you shrug your shoulders? Can you keep it still?
- Can you feel how your hands move up and down when you are performing the movement in tall kneeling?
- Can you feel how the weight shifts across the elbows as you perform the movement in a forearms and knees position?
- Are you breathing?
- When your forearms are on the floor, can you keep your torso up, away from the floor?

STANDING HIP FLEXION WITH ANKLE MOBILITY

Come into a standing position, facing a firm surface that's lower than waist high. Place your right foot on the surface with your right knee straight. If your balance feels tippy, place a dowel in each hand and press the dowels down into the floor for support. Find the triangle of the left foot and reach it into the floor so the foot can support you. The left knee will be straight and strong.

Reach the right toes away from you; the right heel will slide towards you. Reach the right toes back towards you; the right heel will slide away from you. Go back and forth four to six times.

On the last one, when the heel is away from you and the toes are pulling back towards the ceiling, hold that position for two breaths. Can you feel the strength of both legs?

Release the leg and switch sides.

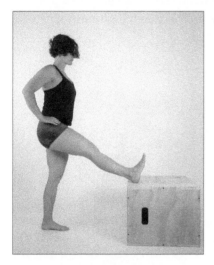 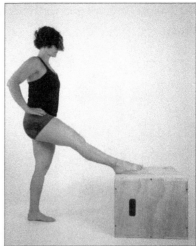

Key Points

- Are the hips square towards the firm surface? If not, can you square them?
- Are the back toes angled out, in, or straight ahead? When you square the hips, does that change the position of the foot?
- Can you keep your jaw relaxed while you press the dowels down?
- Do you lean back, or does your torso stay vertical? If you feel like you are leaning back, can you adjust the weight forward so you are more upright?
- Is one side easier than the other?

CERVICAL PROTRACTION AND RETRACTION, LATERAL FLEXION

Come into a comfortable seated position, either on the floor or on a chair. Make sure you can feel the base of your pelvis against the surface, and if you are seated in a chair, feel your feet against the floor.

Place your left hand on top of your right hand, with your left fingers pointing towards the right and your right fingers pointing towards the left. Place your hands beneath your chin, as though they were making a shelf.

Slide the chin back across the hands and slide the chin forward across the hands. Go back and forth between these two positions four to six times.

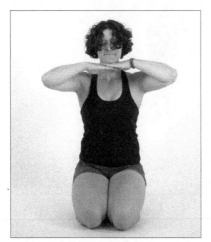 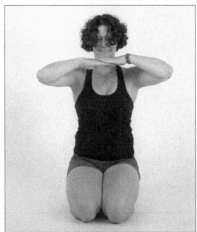

Keeping the chin against the hands, tilt the right ear towards the right shoulder. Bring it to center. Tilt the left ear towards the left shoulder. Go back and forth between the two sides, alternating the movement six to eight times. Relax and rest your hands by your sides.

Key Points

- Keep the movement small and easy. There is no need to strain.
- When you slide the chin back, can you feel motion in the upper spine? What about when you slide it forward?
- Are you able to breathe?
- Is one motion easier than the other?

SEATED SHOULDER STRETCH

Come into a seated position on the floor with your knees bent, your feet flat on the floor, and your hands behind you. Press your hands into the floor, feeling how they support you. Make sure your feet make firm contact with the floor, so they support you as well.

Move your shoulders back, pressing your shoulder blades together. Relax, allowing your shoulders to return to the starting position. Go back and forth between these two positions four to six times.

On your last one, keep the shoulders back and the shoulder blades moving towards each other for two breaths.

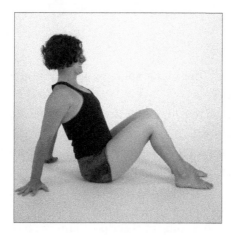

Key Points

- Are you remembering to actively press the hands down the entire time?
- Does your neck change positions, or do your neck and spine stay relatively still while your shoulders move?
- Are you able to breathe?

QUADRUPED TO BENT-KNEE OVERHEAD POSITION

Come into a quadruped position. Actively press the hands into the floor so the knees float off the ground. Keep the knees bent and reach the arms long as you shift the torso back towards the thighs.

Go back and forth between these two positions four to six times, exploring the sensation of pressing the arms overhead while the hands are fixed.

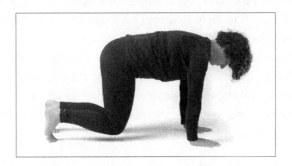

Key Points

- As you shift, does your spine or pelvis round or arch? Can you keep it still?
- As you reach the arms overhead, do you feel the shoulder blades changing position to support you? If not, can you think about what the shoulder blades might do to support the arms overhead?
- Are you remembering to breathe?

You might notice that some of these positions are more active and feel more like strength work. That's because mobility and strength aren't separate; you need both to be able to support the body in new positions. Gently exposing the physical body to new positions gives it time to adjust to what is being asked of it; holding the new position for one or two breaths in an active way creates muscular contraction, which, remember, influences proprioception.

Spend a few minutes reflecting on how you can add variation to these movements. Jot down your ideas and try them out. Below is a quick list of some of the ways I might introduce variation:

- Quadruped Spinal Circles: Lower to the forearm on one side; keep the other hand flat but allow the elbow to bend.
- Split-Stance Hip Shift: Make the legs wider. Reach the arm in different directions, not just straight back and forward.

- Shoulder Shrugs, Two Ways: Alternate the shoulders instead of doing them at the same time.
- Standing Hip Flexion with Ankle Mobility: Rotate the hips away from the firm surface, or rotate the hips more towards the firm surface.
- Cervical Protraction and Retraction, Lateral Flexion: Perform this standing, place the other hand on top.
- Seated Shoulder Stretch: Orient the fingers in a different direction.
- Quadruped to Bent-Knee Overhead Position: Stagger the hands.

Mobility Sequence IV: Dynamic Flexion and Rotation

For this practice, you will need two yoga blocks and a blanket, pillow, or bolster.

SEATED SPINAL FLEXION

Come into a seated position on a firm chair or box. Place your forearms on your thighs.

Round your back towards the ceiling. Move your back away from the ceiling. Go back and forth between these two positions four times. Keep your forearms connected to your thighs the entire time.

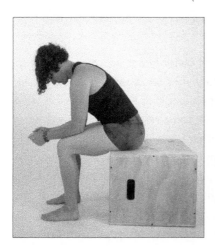
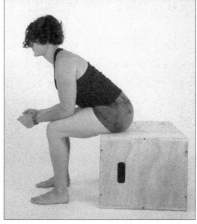

After your fourth one, rest and come into an upright position. Feel the sitting bones against the surface and the feet flat against the floor.

Place the forearms back on the thighs. This time, as you round your back, allow the thighs to come towards each other (so the thighs and forearms move towards each other) and as you arch your back, allow the thighs to move away from each other. Go back and forth between these two positions four times, feeling how your thighs move in and out as you round and arch your back.

Rest in an upright position for two or three breaths.

Bring the forearms back to the thighs and round and arch your back, this time keeping the thighs still. On your fourth one, keep the spine rounded and take two breaths. Imagine that you are filling the space between your shoulder blades with air. Relax after your last breath.

Key Points

- Is there movement throughout the thoracic spine, or does one portion flex more than the other?
- Does the movement become more integrated and fluid as you move through the different variations?
- Which variation is easiest?
- Do your feet stay against the floor the entire time?
- Can you feel the breath move across the middle back?

SIDE-LYING HIP MOBILITY

Lie on your left side, with a pillow or bolster under your head and your knees bent and in front of you. Allow your left shoulder to be on the floor, stacked under the body, if possible. If that isn't comfortable, find a position that allows your upper back to be relatively in line with your pelvis, not rotated one way or the other.

Place your right hand on the top of your right pelvis. Use the right hand to move the right side of the pelvis down towards the right foot. Use the right hand to move the right side of the pelvis up towards the right ribs.

Go back and forth between these two positions four to six times.

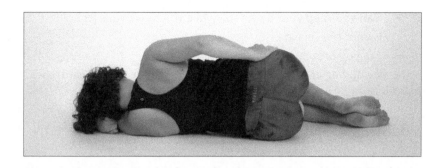

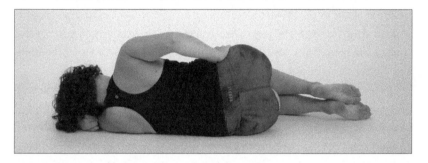

Find a place where the right side of the pelvis feels even with the left side of the pelvis. Reach the right leg straight out, so it is in line with the pelvis (not in front of it or behind it). Bring the right leg forward and backward four to six times. If it's helpful, keep the right hand on the right pelvis so it doesn't move.

Once you have finished moving the leg forward and back, move it up towards the ceiling and back to its starting place. Do this four to six times.

On your last one, keep the leg reaching towards the ceiling (the pelvis should still be in the original starting place). Rotate the right leg so the toes rotate towards the ceiling. Rotate the right leg so the toes point towards the floor. Go back and forth between these two positions four to six times.

If you can maintain the position of the pelvis, make four circles with your right leg going forward. Make four with your right leg going backward.

Switch sides, and perform the same sequence with your left leg.

Key Points

- Is one side easier than the other?

- Can you keep your pelvis still while you move your leg?
- Is your jaw relaxed?
- Are you breathing?
- Is your leg actually in line with your pelvis, or is it forward/back?

WRIST EXTENSION AND AXIAL SHOULDER ROTATION

Stand facing a wall. Place your right hand on the wall so your fingers are pointing straight up towards the ceiling and your right elbow is straight. Rotate your torso to the left. Keep the right arm straight as you rotate. Rotate the torso back towards the wall. Rotate four to six times, keeping the elbow straight and actively pressing the hand into the wall.

After your last one, pause with your torso rotated away from the wall and your right arm straight. Change the hand position so your right hand makes a fist and the fist is reaching into the wall with the thumb oriented towards the ceiling. Rotate the arm so the thumb rotates behind you. Rotate the arm so the thumb rotates down towards the floor. Go back and forth between these two positions four to six times.

Switch sides, and perform the entire sequence on the other side.

Key Points

- When you rotate, can you actively press the wall away from you?
- Does the shoulder move towards the ear as you rotate away from the wall?
- Is one side easier than the other?
- Are you breathing?
- When you rotate the fist, can you feel movement up through your shoulder, or does it mostly happen in the forearm?

ANKLE MOBILITY THROUGH STEPPING

Begin in standing. Keep your torso long, bend your knees, and slide your hands over your knees. (Your butt goes back and down, as if you were sitting in a bucket.)

Peel your right foot off the ground and step it forward. Peel your left foot off the ground and step it forward. Alternate between the two legs, stepping one forward and then the other, feeling how each foot peels off the floor.

Key Points

- When you peel your foot off the floor, does the inside ankle bone move towards or away from the floor?
- Can you feel the weight across the ball of the foot as the foot lifts off the ground?
- Does your knee rotate forward as the heel begins to lift off the floor?
- Is one side easier than the other?
- Does your torso remain long, or do you extend your knees or round your spine as you walk forward? Can you perform the movement in a way in which the spine doesn't change shape as you step forward?
- Are you breathing?

SEATED OPEN-CHAIN ANKLE MOBILITY

Come into a seated position on the floor or on a blanket, bolster, or pillow, with your legs long in front of you. Bend your right knee so your right foot is standing on the floor, and place your hands around your right leg to help keep your torso upright.

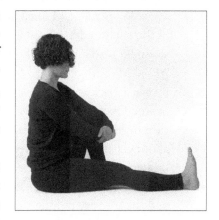

Actively point the left toes away from you. Really think about pointing the toes as much as you can. Feel how the left heel slides towards you as the left toes point away from you. Now pull the toes actively towards the ceiling. The left heel will move away from you as the toes move towards the ceiling.

Go back and forth between these two positions six to eight times. Switch sides.

Key Points

- Can you keep your torso upright as you flex and extend the foot?
- Does your foot cramp when you actively point the toes? (Cramping isn't bad. It's beneficial to observe and see if it improves over time.)
- Can you feel the foot on the side of the bent knee and the pelvis against the floor?
- Are you breathing?

Spend a few minutes reflecting on how you can add variation to these movements. Jot down your ideas and try them out. Below is a quick list of some of the ways I might introduce variation.

- Seated Spinal Flexion: Move one block closer to the body and one block further away so the arms are staggered.
- Side-Lying Hip Mobility: Perform the same sequence with the top knee bent rather than extended.
- Wrist Extension and Axial Shoulder Rotation: Angle the fingers of the anchored hand out (or in). Initiate axial rotation from the shoulder blade instead of the shoulder. How does that feel?
- Ankle Mobility through Stepping: Walk in a variety of ways: forward, backward, sideways, rotating, etc.
- Seated Open-Chain Ankle Mobility: Add an isometric contraction or leg lift in each position (so when the toes point, think about getting as strong as possible in the extended leg and either imagine that you are going to lift the leg off the floor or actually lift the leg off the floor. Do the same thing when the foot is flexed and the toes are pulling back towards the knee).

Mobility Sequence V: Mobility Meets Movement
For this practice, you will need a yoga block or small rubber ball.

LATERAL SPINAL FLEXION IN TALL KNEELING

Come into a tall kneeling position. Place your left palm on your breastbone and your right hand over your left hand. Tilt your breastbone to the left. Bring it back to center. Tilt it to the right. Go back and forth between the two positions six to eight times.

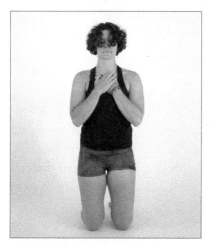 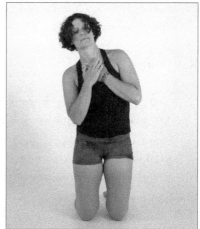

Key Points

- Can you keep your jaw relaxed?
- Do the shoulders tip straight down, remaining in the frontal plane, or do they veer forward or backward? Can you do the movement without them rotating?
- Are you breathing?
- What happens if you think about anchoring the knees into the floor? Does that change your experience?

PRONE SHOULDER MOBILITY WITH BLOCK OR BALL

Lie down on your stomach with your left hand under your forehead and the block or ball on the ground above your right shoulder and slightly to the right. Your right arm will be extended overhead on the floor with the pinkie side of the hand standing on the ground.

Begin reaching the right arm long. As you reach, see if you can feel it beginning to lift off the ground. As it lifts, move it over the block or ball, setting it on the ground next to the block or ball. Begin reaching again, lifting it back up, and bringing it back over the block or ball.

Perform this three or four times, and then move the block or ball to a slightly different location. Try it in the new location three or four times, and then move it one more time to a slightly different location for another three or four repetitions.

When you have finished, do the same thing on the other side.

Key Points

- Do you feel shifting in your torso or pelvis when you lift your arm? Can you keep your pelvis and torso still as you lift and move your arm? (If you are struggling with this, exaggerate the movement, allowing the pelvis and torso to move a few times and then try and keep them still.)
- Are you breathing?
- Does your pubic bone feel like it rests evenly on the floor, or does it rotate to one side? If it feels rotated or you are unable to feel the pelvis against the ground, place a small bolster or blanket under your pelvis as you perform the movement. See if that helps.
- Can you feel the reaching action before you lift?
- Is one side easier than the other?

KNEE CIRCLES

Come into a standing position. Place your hands on your knees with your knees bent. Begin drawing circles with your knees.

Draw four circles going in one direction and then reverse the direction for four more circles.

Key Points

- Can you feel the change in pressure across your feet as you draw circles with your knees?
- Is one direction easier than the other?

- What happens if you take your hands off your knees? Can you still make the circular motion?

UPRIGHT SQUAT TO HEEL RAISE VARIATION I

Come into a standing position with your feet under your hips. Reach your arms forward and maintain an upright torso as you bend your knees, keeping your heels on the ground.

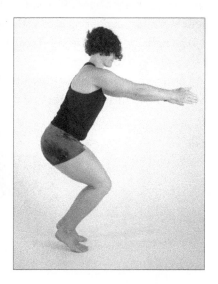

When your knees can no longer bend, lift your heels off the ground, keeping your torso still (your head will not move closer to the ceiling). Lower your heels back down. Perform this four to six times.

When you finish, rest for a moment, and then perform the same action, while allowing the head to move closer towards the ceiling when the heels lift. Does that feel different?

Key Points

- When you lift the heels, is the weight even across the feet, or do you roll to the outside or the inside of the feet? Play with the weight distribution and see what it's like to allow the weight to be even across the feet.
- Are you breathing?
- Do your knees remain pointed in the same direction when you lift your heels, or do they shift in or out? Can you keep them pointing straight ahead?

CRAWL TO LUNGE ROTATION

Come into a quadruped position, with your hands under your shoulders and your knees under your hips or a little behind them.

Float your knees off the ground and step your right foot forward, next to your right hand. Pick your right hand up off the ground as your foot steps forward, bring it to your chest, and allow your torso to rotate to the right. Your back leg (left leg) will naturally straighten as your hand lifts and torso rotates.

Bring your hand back down to the floor as your foot steps back. Switch sides; this completes one round. Perform four to six rounds.

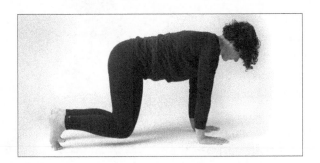

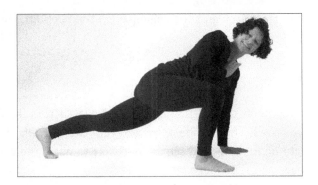

Key Points

- Can you feel strong contact with your hand against the floor?
- What does your head do when your torso rotates? Does it rotate with your torso?
- Is one side easier than the other?
- Are you breathing?

Spend a few minutes reflecting on how you can add variation to these movements. Jot down your ideas and try them out. Below are some of the ways I might introduce variation.

SEATED LATERAL SPINAL FLEXION

Sit down on the floor or on a folded blanket or pillow. Start with your legs in a wide straddle. Bend your left leg in, placing the left foot against the right inner thigh.

Place your left hand on the floor, slightly away from your left hip. Lean your weight into your left hand as you bring your right hand to your chest.

Transfer weight away from your left hand, bringing your left hand behind your head as you reach your right forearm to your right thigh. Imagine the left elbow is going to touch the ceiling.

Move back and forth between the two positions, pausing occasionally to breathe.

Key Points

- Keep the ribs soft.
- Make sure you are side bending, not side shifting.
- Keep your eyes following the trajectory of the elbow that's moving towards the ceiling.
- Is one side easier than the other?
- Are you breathing?

PRONE SHOULDER MOBILITY

Lie on your stomach with your arms extended out in a "T" position. Place your left hand under your left shoulder and look to your left.

Press your left hand into the floor as you bring your left leg away from the floor and your left foot behind your right leg. You will roll on to your right side as your left foot comes to the floor and your left knee points towards the ceiling.

Return to the starting position. Perform four to six times and switch sides.

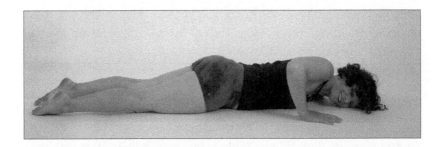

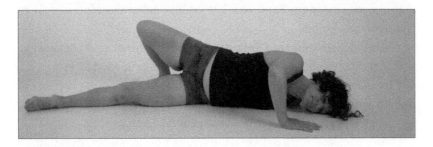

Key Points

- Be sure to actively press your arm and hand into the floor on the side you are rolling away from.
- Are you breathing?
- Is one side easier than the other?

Variation

- Try placing your arm at slightly different heights. How does that change things?

QUADRUPEDAL INTERNAL AND EXTERNAL ROTATION

Come into a quadruped position with your hands under your shoulder and your knees under your hips. Place a rolled-up towel or tennis ball at the outside of your right lower leg.

Lift your right lower leg up off the floor and over the towel or tennis ball. Return your leg to the starting position. Your right knee stays on the floor.

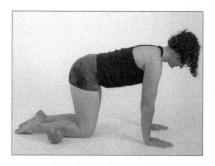 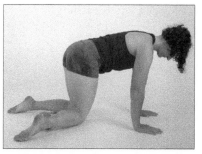

Go back and forth, lifting your right lower leg up and over the tennis ball or towel and then returning to the starting position four to six times. After you have finished, switch sides.

Key Points

- Are you able to clear the object with your lower leg?
- Is one side easier than the other?
- Are you breathing?

Variation

- Place the knees closer together or further apart while lifting the lower leg over the towel or ball.

UPRIGHT SQUAT TO HEEL RAISE VARIATION II

Come into a standing position with your feet under your hips and your toes pointing straight ahead. Keep your torso upright and your heels on the floor as you bend your knees.

With your knees bent and your torso upright, lift your left heel off the floor. Lower it down as you lift the right heel off the floor. Perform this four to six times on each side and then lower your heels and straighten your knees to return to the starting position.

Key Points

- Are you able to keep your torso upright?
- Are you able to keep your ribs soft?

- Are you breathing?

Variation

- Start with both heels lifted. Stagger the feet.

The five mobility sequences above move from simple to more complex in terms of mobility demands and effort required to perform the movements. These are just ideas—once you understand the principles, you can sequence things in a wide variety of ways.

References

Blum K.P., Lamotte D'Incamps B., Zytnicki D., & Ting L.H. (2017). Force encoding in muscle spindles during stretch of passive muscle. PLOS Computer Biology, 13(9), 1-24.

Colon A., Guo X., Akanda N., Cai Y., & Hickman J.J. (2017). Functional analysis of human intrafusal fiber innervation by human γ-motoneurons. Scientific Reports, 7, 17202.

Cuoco A., & Tyler T.F. (2012). Chapter 26: Plyometric Training and Drills, 571-595. In: Andrews J.R., Harrelson G.L., & Wilk K.E. (eds) Physical Rehabilitation of the Injured Athlete. 4th edition. Cambridge, MA: Elsevier.

Edwards L.L., King E.M., Buetefisch C.M., & Borich M.R. (2019). Putting the "sensory" into sensorimotor control: The role of sensorimotor integration in goal-directed hand movements after stroke. Frontiers in Integrative Neuroscience, 13, 16.

Greene E., & Goodrich-Dunn (2004). The Psychology of the Body. 2nd edition. Philadelphia, PA: Lippincott Williams & Wilkins.

Law R.W.A., Harvey L.A., Nicholas M.K., Tonkin L., De Sousa M., & Finnis D.G. (2009). Stretch exercises increase tolerance to stretch in patients with chronic musculoskeletal pain: A randomized controlled trial. Physical Therapy, 89(10), 1016-1026.

Main C.J., Buchbinder R., Pocheret M., & Foster N. (2010). Addressing patient beliefs and expectations in the consultation. Best Practice and Research Clinical Rheumatology, 24(2), 219-225.

Page P. (2012). Current concepts in muscle stretching for exercise and rehabilitation. International Journal of Sports Physical Therapy, 7(1), 109-119.

Smith D.L., & Plowman S.A. (2006). Chapter 2: Understanding Muscle Contraction, 369-379. In: Donatelli R. (ed.) Sport-Specific Rehabilitation. Churchill Livingston: London.

Weppler C.H., & Magnusson S.P. (2010). Increasing muscle extensibility: A matter of increasing length or modifying sensation? Physical Therapy, 3(1), 438-449.

CHAPTER 9

Mindful Movement
and Play

"Can I try it again?"

"Of course."

"I think I can get it this time."

The client is a 75-year-old with chronic low back pain and mild depression. He is bouncing a ball with his left hand while tossing another ball with his right hand. The coordination is throwing him off a little bit, but he is moving quickly, trying different techniques, and is focused on achieving a string of successful attempts.

This type of work focuses his attention. It's interesting for him and gives him a moment where he isn't focused on his discomfort. He moves in a much less guarded, more varied way when he is performing these types of tasks, and when he finishes, I can see the shift in his mood. The task does more than improve his hand-eye coordination—it's an entry point to connecting his mind with his body.

One way to implement mindful movement into a practice is through playful techniques that focus attention outside of the self. Remember that I am defining mindful movement as breathing, grounding, centering, and listening; externally focused game play requires listening with all of the senses, which conveniently results in grounding/centering (depending on the skill that is being learned).

I mentioned breath holding, a strategy people use when they are first exposed to dynamic balance work or new and challenging situations, earlier. Breath holding is not always necessary, and reminding people to check in periodically with their breath can help them notice the difference between breathing and not breathing. At the end of the chapter, some of the exercises draw attention to whether you are breathing or how you are breathing. You can also do breath-centered work for individuals for whom the breath isn't anxiety provoking.

Play versus Work

The definition of play is up for debate, though it is becoming evident that play throughout the lifespan is important for lifelong learning and curiosity. Researchers agree that play, like many of the concepts discussed throughout this book, exists across a spectrum. There is free play, which is play without guidance or support. This is what your three-year-old does when she is outside in the garden with two toys, a shovel, and no one telling her what she should or shouldn't do.

At the other end of the spectrum are guided play and games, which involve general rules and support while keeping a playful element. The activity I used with my 75-year-old client above is an example of guided play—I provided the rules for the task and the client interpreted those rules to accomplish the task. It is exceptionally rare to see adults participating in free play. (When was the last time you picked up an object and began exploring what you could do with it, making up a story behind it in your head? I am guessing it's probably been a while.) In a movement context, play is usually governed by constraints and a loose task that can be accomplished in several different ways. Play is generally defined as an activity done for its own sake, without a specific end goal. The process is the interesting piece, the piece that keeps people trying even after you have said that it is time to move on to something else (Zosh *et al.*, 2018).

Play differs from exploration, which is considered a focused investigation on something new, like an object or new environment. Play often begins with exploration; then, when the curiosity in an object or environment sparks an idea, a thought of "What if I try and get under this rail that's thick, sturdy, and low?" the idea turns into an act that is performed repeatedly and never in the same way, captivating attention and causing time to disappear. Play may be the outcome of exploration, but it isn't a guaranteed outcome (again, especially as adults—we all know when we walk into someone's house for the first time, we aren't supposed to pick up objects, inspect them, and decide how they could be used to create an intricate crawling game).

Work, which has a goal, can be used to facilitate play in a movement setting. For instance, the four sets of deadlifts I did this morning at about a 65 percent intensity level were performed for reps, had a purpose (maintain strength and load the tissues on the posterior side of my body), and were done in a defined way (barbell deadlifts, conventional grip, for reps). Though you can definitely use play to build strength, at some point, depending on your goals, a certain amount of work is required to give you more options for how you play, whether it's through the development of strength, power, flexibility, or some combination of the three.

Games also differ from play in that there is a goal or desired outcome that usually involves a judgment of performance. When you play someone in a friendly tennis match, there are defined rules and constraints that allow you to determine whether you are winning or losing. The act of play occurs during practice to explore new ways of improving ball skills or discover new ways of moving. This can have far-reaching benefits, especially if it challenges the learner in some way and allows an interaction between information processing, having clear task demands, and practice. The lessons learned during playful practice carry over to improved options during game play and can result in a more skilled player (Zeng *et al.*, 2017; Sullivan *et al.*, 2008).

Though most of the research on play is done in children, many of the concepts related to the benefits of play can be applied to adults in movement settings. Adults, like children, benefit from creative thinking and allowing movement to be flexible. Rather than structured sets and reps, play allows the client to meet the needs of the task in an inquisitive, undefined way (Russ & Wallace, 2013). This differs from traditional exercise classes and settings, where adults are told how to move their bodies and where to place their limbs.

Coaching individuals on how to move efficiently is tremendously valuable and leads to improved skill development and the ability to generate power effectively. But introducing movement problem solving that emphasizes creativity, spontaneity, curiosity, and pleasure has tremendous carry-over, not just in how individuals relate to movement, but also in how they perceive and evaluate situations outside of the gym (Guitard *et al.*, 2005).

The ability to master new skills requires the resolution of motor redundancy (Rohde *et al.*, 2019). When you approach a new task, the sensorimotor system has to choose from several different ways to achieve the goal. In play-based tasks that have constraints, the sensorimotor system first determines which options are available and then chooses which one will most effectively accomplish the task. One of the things that happens in adults who don't move regularly is they forget there are multiple ways to perform the same task.

When I do agility training with my puppy, sometimes I ask her to go over objects that she deems not good for going over. Instead, she will go under or around them. When she is left to her own devices, she experiments with different paths over, around, and under objects of various sizes and heights. When we play together, she draws from previously performed movements to determine the best solution for the task at hand (which sometimes isn't my solution).

This is the benefit of spending a few minutes regularly exploring movement in an unstructured way. Sometimes you stumble upon things that work well in a different setting or feel interesting in that moment. These small discoveries can lead to more interest in movement in general, which leads to more movement being incorporated into a person's daily life.

TRY THIS: Set a timer for three minutes. Sit on the floor. Stand up from the floor. Notice how you did it. Sit back down on the floor a different way. Stand up a different way. Get up and down from the floor in as many ways as you can think of until the timer goes off. Try to make each sequence of getting up and getting down different than the ones you have done previously.

What limits a person's ability to come up with different ways to get up and down off the floor? A lack of creativity or experience playing with movement in this way, is a limiting factor. Another thing that limits options is mobility. While it could be argued that performing a task like this will improve mobility over time (and it will), I find that spending time working on mobility for a few weeks before asking someone to perform this type of task is more rewarding for the individual. When someone is asked to perform a task that makes them self-conscious because they don't feel "good" at it, or they lack the options available to complete the task in a way they deem successful, the exploration becomes less playful and more stressful. I like to set clients up to be as successful as possible; adequate mobility for getting up and down off the floor makes the task more interesting because it is more achievable.

Creativity, Constraints, and Learning

Learning to problem solve with a specific set of constraints introduces variable movement. In the activity above, you used the constraint of standing up and sitting down differently each time. When we discussed variable movement in Chapter 4, we looked at improving strength and loading the tissues. Moving in a variety of ways is also effective for improving range of motion or mobility. While motor tasks that resemble play aren't necessarily performed to improve strength or mobility, the outcome generally results in novel movement patterns. This often leads to an increase in both strength and mobility.

The Value of Constraints

In 1909, Hermann Munk, a German scientist, came up with the concept of constraint-induced movement therapy (CIMT) when he noticed that primates who had sensation cut off to one of their upper limbs would use that limb in purposeful movement when other options weren't available (Kwakkel *et al.*, 2015). More recent studies showed that monkeys who have had sensation cut off in a limb won't use the impaired limb unless specific scenarios are set up that teach them how to overcome their preference and use the injured limb (*ibid.*).

CIMT eventually found its way into rehabilitation settings for neurological conditions and is frequently used in stroke rehabilitation programs. It consists of three main components.

The first is practicing a task that uses the affected limb in a specific way. The task becomes more challenging as the affected limb becomes more capable, so the limb continues to get stronger.

Imagine that you don't feel like you have a lot of control over your right arm. It's difficult to move and you don't use it during your everyday life. One way to introduce a task-based movement for the right arm might be to place three glasses relatively close to and in front of you and sit on your left hand. You could then pick up each glass with your right hand and set it back down. Once this is comfortable, you could set the glasses up a bit further apart and to your left and right and at the center of your body, and repeat the exercise. You could vary this in several ways: by doing the same thing with the glasses set at different levels, by standing or sitting at different heights, and by changing the glasses around so they are in different configurations.

The second component is constraining the non-affected limb. The suggestion above to sit on the left hand is an example of constraining the non-affected limb. If you kept your left hand in your pocket all day and forced yourself to use your right hand to perform all of your daily movements, there would be a shift in your perception (and use) of your right hand.

Finally, the third component is using specifically designed adherence-enhancing behavioral methods to transfer clinical gains to a real-world environment. Creating a positive feedback loop when you use the right hand, by using a reward or by making daily movements into a game where you see how many ways you can use the right hand to accomplish specific tasks, can increase adherence by making you feel confident and successful.

Obviously, the goals behind a general movement program that promotes emotional and physical well-being are different than the goals for stroke rehabilitation. What they do have in common is creating experiences that use the whole self. We all have movement habits. The stronger the habit, the more rigid we become in our movement pathways. Adding constraints forces us to confront our habits. As a result, we search for a way to achieve the task using movements or ranges of motion that are unfamiliar. The more we confront our habits and our preferences, the more adaptable we become, in all aspects of our life.

The idea of using graded practice in CIMT should, at this point, seem like a familiar motor control, strength, and mobility concept. I mentioned above that one of the limitations to getting up from and down to the floor in a variety of ways is lack of options due to limited range of motion. For the individual who is unable to get down to the floor comfortably, getting up and down in novel ways might not be a good choice. It's too complex, both physically and from a problem-solving standpoint. Instead, a good coach would regress the constraint so the client can achieve the task most of the time. The client should feel challenged but not so challenged that they never succeed. The task also shouldn't be so easy that they easily succeed and become bored. Learning researchers call this sweet spot of difficulty the "Goldilocks zone," where motivation and learning are optimized (Wilson *et al.*, 2019). (Researchers have actually quantified the ideal failure rate at 15 percent, meaning that succeeding 85 percent of the time and failing the rest of the time results in exponential improvements in the rate of learning (*ibid.*).)

This means that when constraints are introduced, they shouldn't make the task feel overwhelmingly difficult. If the goals are to focus attention, keep the participant engaged while improving motor control, and introduce variability and creative problem solving into the participant's movement repertoire, the task needs to be appropriate for the individual.

The science of learning and development (SoLD) is a recent synthesis of educational research that blends evidence from biology, neurology, sociology, psychology, and learning sciences to promote a child's well-being, healthy development, and transferable learning. SoLD concludes that the activation of the neural networks involved in learning is dependent on experience and influenced by what's happening physically, cognitively, and/or affectively. What children experience emotionally or socially can impact attention, concentration, and memory, just like what children experience physically can impact how they feel emotionally (Darling-Hammond *et al.*, 2020).

Adult learning functions in much the same way. When the environment feels safe, there is social support, and curiosity is fostered through appropriate physical challenges, people thrive. The rest of this chapter is devoted to ideas for fostering grounding, centering, and appropriate task-based challenges that are playful in nature.

Mindful Movement and Play Practice I: A Standing Practice

For this practice, you will need four yoga blocks or like-sized objects.

GROUNDING THE FEET PART I

Begin in a standing position, with your feet about hip distance apart and your arms relaxed by your sides. Rock onto your heels, allowing the front of the feet to lift. Rock onto the front of the feet, allowing the heels to lift. Go back and forth between these two positions eight to ten times.

When you finish, find a position that feels centered. Take two breaths, feeling the feet against the floor.

Key Points

- Is it easier to rock backward or forward?

- Does the torso move as a unit, or does it break? (Another way to think of this is: does half the torso bend forward while half bends back or vice versa?)

GROUNDING THE FEET PART II

Remain in a standing position with your feet about hip distance apart. Rock to the right, allowing the feet to respond to the weight shift (the left foot might begin to lift away from the floor). Rock to the left, allowing the right foot to lift away from the floor. Shift your weight from right to left eight to ten times, feeling how the feet respond to the movement.

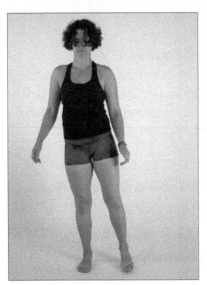 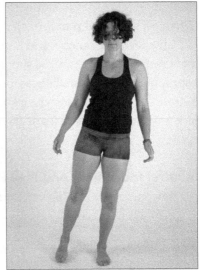

When you have finished, come into a comfortable standing position for two to four breaths. Feel the weight of your feet against the floor. Does it feel like the weight is evenly distributed between the right and left foot? Or does one feel heavier than the other?

Key Points

- Is it easier to rock to the right or to the left? Or is the experience fairly balanced?

- Does the torso easily respond to the movement and rock to the left or right?
- Where is the gaze?

PAINTING THE FENCE

Begin in a comfortable standing position with your arms by your sides and your hands relaxed. Raise your arms. Imagine that you are painting a fence directly in front of you with an upward stroke. At the top of the fence, imagine that you are painting the fence in front of you with a downward stroke—you will be making a repeated up-and-down motion, gradually moving up and then down again. The wrists will respond to the movement of the arms. Perform this three times.

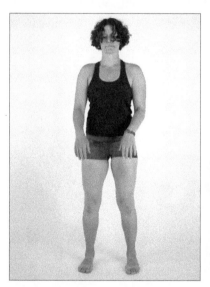 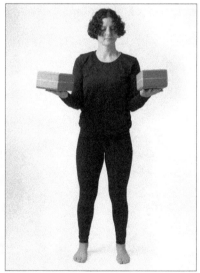

After your third round, see if you can match the breath to the arm movement. Try inhaling as the arm raises and exhaling as the arm lowers. Perform this three times. Now try exhaling as the arm raises and inhaling as the arm lowers. Perform this three times.

After your last one, pause. Feel the sensation of your arms by your sides as you gently breathe.

Key Points

- Do the elbows stay relatively straight during the movement?
- Does it make more sense to inhale while the arms are lifting or while they are lowering?
- Does the torso stay relatively stable during the movement?
- Is it easier to extend the wrist or flex the wrist?

TEACUPS VARIATION I

Set a timer for two minutes. Place a yoga block in each hand, with the palms facing up towards the ceiling. Without letting the blocks fall, move the blocks in front of your body, behind the body, overhead, out to the sides, across the body... Move the blocks in as many different ways you can think of, either together or individually.

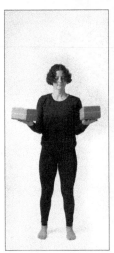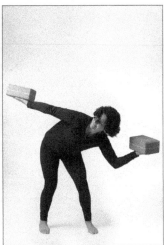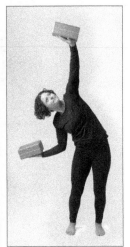

Constraints

- Keep the feet in contact with the floor the entire time (the heels can lift, but the forefoot should remain connected). The knees can bend and the torso can shift.
- Keep the palms flat.
- Don't let the blocks fall.

Key Points

- Can you feel the body respond to the task of moving the blocks?
- Is there a position you are unable to achieve? What prevents you from moving into the position (maybe you don't know how to accomplish it successfully, you are limited by discomfort, lack of mobility, or something else)?
- Do you repeat the same pattern several times? If so, why? Does it feel good, is it familiar, do you know you can succeed?

HEEL-TO-TOE WALKING

Note: If you don't feel comfortable with one foot directly in front of the other, place yourself near a wall so your fingers can lightly graze the wall as needed.

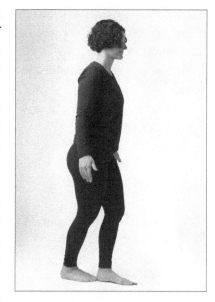

Begin in a comfortable standing position. Look around the room, identifying objects on the walls and ceiling you can easily see, allowing your head to turn.

Pick an object on the wall or ceiling in front of you. As you look ahead, place your right heel in front of your left foot, in line with your left toes.

Shift your gaze to another part of the room and step your left heel in front of your right toes.

Perform this pattern for eight to ten steps. Shift your gaze each time you take a step.

When you finish, pause and observe your balance in quiet standing.

Key Points

- Are you remembering to breathe?

- Do you find yourself focusing on the same thing? Why? Is it visually pleasing, comfortable, or something else?
- Do you shift your gaze while stepping, before stepping, or after stepping?
- Is there any aspect of the movement that you are rushing (such as switching from the left to right foot or shifting your gaze from left to right or up to down)?

REACHING FROM STANDING VARIATION I

Begin standing. Stack the four yoga blocks so they are next to your right leg. Reach your left hand across your body to take the top block and set it somewhere on the floor. You can set it on the floor in front of you, to the left of you, next to the stack of blocks, behind you... Set it wherever you think is interesting.

Repeat this with your left hand until all of the blocks have been placed on the floor.

Pick up one block at a time with the left hand and stack them next to the left foot.

Repeat with the right hand.

Constraints

- Keep the feet in contact with the floor (the heels can lift as needed).
- The blocks can't be placed right next to each other.

Key Points

- Do you stand up between each reach, or do you stay bent over the entire time?
- Is one side easier than the other?
- Is there a position you are avoiding (for instance, placing the block behind you)?
- Do you prefer to set the blocks close to the body, far away from the body, or a bit of both?

Mindful Movement and Play Practice II:
A Floor-Based Practice

For this practice, you will need a light medicine ball (of four to eight pounds) or a small rubber ball. The type of ball you use doesn't really matter; if you have access to both, try them and see how they feel.

ROCKING

Begin on your hands and knees with your hands under your shoulders and your knees under your hands. Rock your belly button back. Rock it forward. Perform this six to eight times.

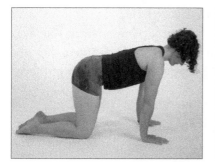 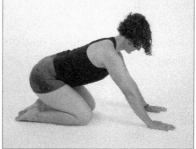

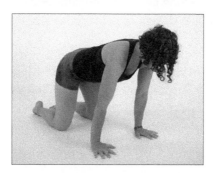

Find center. Rock your torso to the right. Rock it to the left. Perform this six to eight times. Return to center. Take two breaths, observing the weight in the hands and in the feet.

Key Points

- Is it easier to rock forward and back or side to side?
- Where is your gaze as you rock? Play with it, looking down, forward, and up. See what feels most natural for you.
- When you rest in the centered position, does it feel like the weight is even in the hands and knees, or does one side feel heavier than the other?

REACHING IN HALF KNEELING

Come into a half kneeling position and move your right foot forward. Begin with your right foot in line with your right hip.

Look around the room, identifying different things to focus your eyes on. You can choose things that are in front of you, down and to the right of you, up and to the left of you, slightly behind you... Allow your eyes to look at a variety of places.

After you have taken in your surroundings, reach your hands towards an object in the room. Really reach for it, as though you were going to touch it. Allow your torso and hips to respond to the movement.

Return to the starting position, and choose a different place in the room to reach for. Do this six to eight times and then switch legs and repeat.

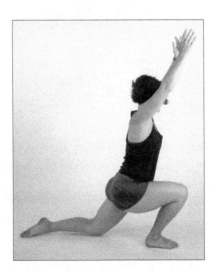

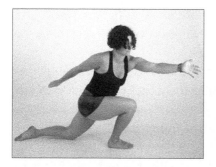 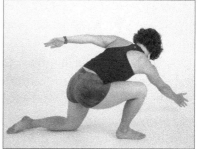

Once you have finished, place your right foot forward again, but place it in a different position (more to the right, more forward, or more to the left). Try the reaching exercise again. See if it feels different with the right foot in a different place. Do this six to eight times and repeat with the left foot forward.

Constraints

- Keep the front heel in contact with the ground the entire time.
- Reach either one or both hands for the object.

Key Points

- Does any position feel particularly interesting?
- Does any position feel particularly challenging?
- Is one side easier than the other?
- Does changing the position of the front foot change the exercise at all?
- Are you remembering to breathe?

SEATED HAND EXPLORATION

Come into a seated position on the floor. Choose a position that's comfortable and that you can stay in for a while (prop yourself up on a blanket or bolster if needed).

Place the palms of your hands together so your fingers are even. Spread your fingers, fanning them out. Bring your fingers back together. Perform this six to eight times.

Now, with the fingers together, move just the third and the fourth fingers away from the center. Bring them back together. Do this six to eight times.

Keep the third and fourth fingers together and move the index fingers and pinkies away from the center. Bring them back together. Do this six to eight times.

Finally, move the index fingers away from each other a few times. Now try the third fingers, then the fourth fingers, then the pinkies, and then the thumbs. After you have played with this, rest your hands by your sides.

Key Points

- Do you find any aspects challenging? Which ones?
- Are you able to keep the palms together the entire time?
- Are you clenching your jaw or holding your breath?

GROUNDED HAND QUADRUPED TRANSITION

- Set a timer for two minutes. Begin in a quadruped position with your hands under your shoulders and your knees under your hips.
- Pick the right hand up and place it on your chest. Keeping your left hand in contact with the floor, move into a different position. Return to quadruped. Move into a different position. Move back to quadruped. Choose different positions to move into until the timer goes off. Reset the timer, switch hands, and do the same thing with the right hand grounded.

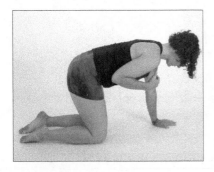 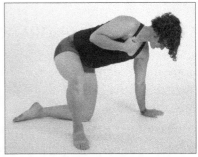

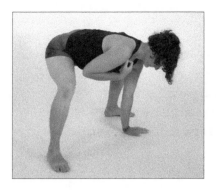

Constraints

- Keep the grounded hand in contact with the floor the entire time.
- Keep the right hand on the chest the entire time.

Key Points

- Does one side feel more comfortable than the other? If so, which one?
- Is it easier to move away from the starting position or move back into the starting position, or does it depend?
- Is there anything you are finding particularly interesting?

QUADRUPED BALL PLAY

Set a timer for three minutes. Begin in a quadruped position with the ball near your left hand. With your left hand, pass the ball to your right hand. Perform this a few times, getting comfortable with what it's like to pass the ball between the hands.

Once you feel comfortable with ball passing, begin passing the ball slightly forward or slightly back, so you have to move to get it. You can make this as challenging or as easy as you would like. For an additional challenge, float the knees off the floor while passing the ball.

When the timer goes off, rest. Observe how you feel.

Constraints

- Keep three limbs in contact with the floor at all times (one hand and two knees or one hand and two feet).
- Moving is allowed. Crawling to reach the ball is perfectly okay.
- You can rebound the ball off a wall if you like.
- You can have a partner pass you the ball.

Key Points

- Choose the variation that appropriately challenges you.
- Rest as needed (three minutes can feel like a long time).
- Do you favor one hand over the other?

Mindful Movement and Play Practice III: A Centering Practice

For this practice you will need one or two dowels.

SPINAL WAVES, TALL KNEELING

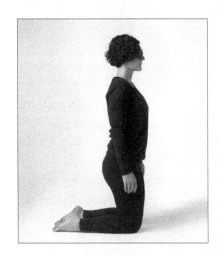

Begin in a tall kneeling position. Imagine that there is a wall half an inch in front of your nose. Move your nose towards the imaginary wall, move your chest towards the imaginary wall, move your belly towards the imaginary wall, and finally, move your pelvis towards the imaginary wall. (If you like, you can orient yourself so you are in front of an actual wall.)

As various parts of your body move towards the wall, other parts will move away from the wall, creating a wave-live motion. Do this six to eight times.

When you finish, pause. Now see if you can initiate the wave from your pelvis, moving your pelvis towards the wall first, and then your belly, chest, and nose. Perform this wave six to eight times. Pause and take two to three breaths, observing the sensation of your spine as you breathe.

Key Points

- As your spine waves, is the movement fluid? Or are there parts of your spine that are more difficult to incorporate into the waving motion than others?
- Do you prefer initiating the movement from the head or the pelvis?
- What happens if you try the same motion standing? Is it easier or more challenging?

FOOT AWARENESS, STANDING

Set a timer for two minutes. Start moving your body in different ways and into different positions but keep part of your right foot connected to the floor at all times. Feel how the weight in the right foot shifts to accommodate the movement. Feel free to change levels by moving towards the floor with your hands or away from the floor with your hands if you find that interesting, or you can stay in an upright position the entire time. The left foot can move freely.

When the timer goes off, pause with both feet on the floor. Does one feel different than the other?

Reset the timer and do the same thing while keeping the left foot connected to the floor at all times.

When you finish, pause for two breaths with your feet even. As you breathe, can you feel the sense of the feet pressing into the floor?

Key Points

- Are there aspects of the foot you avoided?
- Which foot feels easier to keep connected?
- When you find center after doing each foot, do you feel equally balanced or does one foot feel more grounded than the other?

DOWEL BALANCE

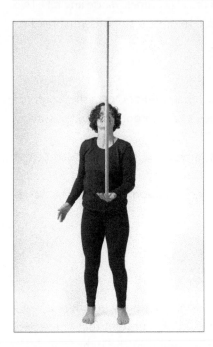

Set a timer for two minutes. Open your right hand and use your left hand to place the end of the dowel in your right palm with the dowel extended straight up towards the ceiling.

Gently let go of the dowel with your left hand and see if you can balance the dowel in your right hand. Move your feet as needed.

When the timer goes off, switch sides.

Key Points

- Touch the dowel with the non-balancing hand as needed to rebalance it.
- Looking up towards the end of the dowel tends to help with balance.
- Don't forget to breathe.

SIDEWAYS BALL-OF-THE-FOOT WALKING

Place the dowel on the floor (if you have two dowels, place the ends together so they make one long line).

Stand facing the dowels with the toes barely touching them. Lift your heels away from the floor. Begin walking sideways along the length of the dowels.

When you get to the end, keep your heels lifted and walk sideways going the other way along the other side of the dowels. Perform two to three laps.

Constraints

- Don't push the dowels forward (they should remain in the same place the entire time).
- Keep the heels lifted the entire time, if possible.

Key Points

- Is one direction easier than the other?
- Are you able to keep the dowels in the same place?
- Are you remembering to breathe?
- Is it easier with the knees bent a little or the knees straight? Try it both ways.
- What are you doing with your hands? Try it with your hands in different places (in front of you with the arms straight or with the elbows bent, arms out to the sides, making fists, with your hands open...).

KINESPHERE PRACTICE

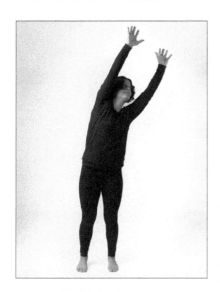

Set a timer for three minutes. Come into a standing position. Imagine that you are in a giant bubble. With your hands, begin reaching towards different places in the bubble. Which places can you reach? Which are more challenging?

After you have explored that for a little while, shift and use your head to reach towards different parts of the bubble. Do this for a while, and then use one of your legs to reach different parts of the bubble. Go slowly, exploring the different aspects of space that you can reach. Place your hands on the floor as needed.

When the timer goes off, pause with your feet centered and breathe for three or four breaths.

Constraints

- When the feet are in contact with the ground, the heels and front of the feet can lift, but they should never rotate.
- Reach as far as you can in any direction without losing your balance.

Key Points

- Are there places you don't explore? Where are they?
- Do you prefer reaching with your hands or your leg?
- Is there an area that feels particularly comfortable or familiar?

Mindful Movement and Play Practice IV: Balance and Centering

This practice requires a yoga block and a narrow surface to balance on, like a very low rail or half foam roller.

LATERAL REACHING IN STANDING

Come into a standing position with your feet comfortably supporting you. Place your fingertips on your shoulders (your elbows will be bent out to the sides).

Tilt your left elbow towards your left foot; allow the left waist to shorten. Return to center. Switch sides, tilting the right elbow towards your right foot.

Go back and forth between these two positions four to six times. When you finish, rest in center.

Begin with your arms by your sides. Slide your left fingertips up towards your left armpit as your right hand slides down towards your right knee. Slide the right hand up towards the right armpit as the left hand slides down towards the left knee. Gently alternate sliding one hand up as the other hand slides down four to six times.

When you finish, rest in a standing position with your hands by your sides for three breaths, observing the feeling of your body.

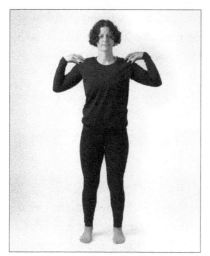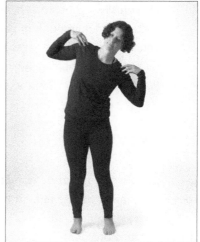

Key Points

- Which variation feels more natural? Why?
- Do your feet remain in contact with the ground the entire time? If not, can you find a way to ground the feet as you laterally flex the spine?
- Does your head respond to the movement? Where do your eyes look? Can you allow your gaze to be soft?
- Are you breathing?

BALANCE ON A LOW RAIL

Set a timer for one minute. Place your left foot on the low rail or half foam roller so it supports the length of the foot. Keep your right toes in contact with the floor.

Begin to play with lifting the right toes away from the floor, allowing the left foot to support you. If this feels scary, keep the right toes on the floor or place yourself next to a wall so your fingers can lightly graze the wall for support. Play with supporting yourself as much as possible on the left foot until the timer goes off. Switch sides.

Key Points

- Are you remembering to breathe?
- Do you allow your arms to respond to the movement or do you try and keep them rigid? It might seem counterintuitive, but allowing your arms and torso to respond in a non-rigid (but stable) way will make the act of balancing in this scenario easier.
- Is one side easier than the other?

TEACUPS VARIATION II

Set a timer for two minutes. Stand and take your legs wide, allowing the toes to turn away as needed. Turn your right palm towards the ceiling and place a light object, such as a yoga block or ball, on it so it lies flat in the palm. Turn the right hand in towards the body, allowing the elbow to move away from the body, and bring the block behind you. Bring it back through to the front and rotate the arm so the block moves away from the body and up and overhead. Begin exploring different ways of moving the right arm, allowing the knees to bend, the heels to lift, and the torso to move in order to accommodate the movement of the arm.

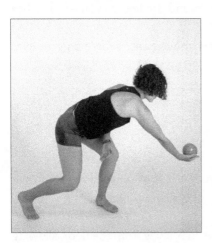 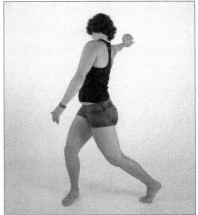

When the timer goes off, switch arms.

When you finish, set the block down and take a moment to breathe three to five times, feeling the weight of your feet on the floor and observing your sense of center.

Constraints

- Keep the feet in contact with the floor the entire time—the heels can lift and rotate.
- Keep the block on the flat palm the entire time.

Key Points

- Is one side easier than the other?
- Are you breathing?
- Does it get easier as you spend time with it?

GROUND TRANSITION, USING THE HAND

Set a timer for two minutes. Begin in a seated position on the floor. Choose whatever position feels most comfortable for you.

While keeping at least one hand in contact with the floor, begin to transition to a standing position. Keep the hand in contact with the floor for as long as possible, lifting it just before you stand up. Move back down to the floor, taking the hand to the floor as soon as possible.

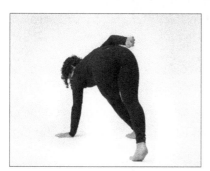
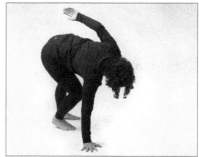

Continue getting up and down off the floor and maintaining as much contact as possible with the hand until the timer goes off.

Constraints

- Keep one hand in contact with the floor for as long as possible (make sure you use both hands).

- Begin in seated and return to seated, using different pathways and explorations.

Key Points

- Do you find yourself defaulting to the same pathway to get up? If so, what limits your exploration?
- Which hand do you prefer to keep in contact with the ground?
- Are you remembering to breathe?

EXPLORING SPACE ON THE FLOOR

Set a timer for three minutes. Lie on your back on a surface on which you can glide (preferably not a carpet or a stick mat). Begin exploring the space around you with your right hand, reaching as far as you can in different directions.

After spending time with your right hand, switch to your left hand, then your right leg, and then your left leg. See if you can spend a bit of time exploring the surrounding area with each limb. You may even try exploring the space with multiple limbs at a time, gliding them against the floor in one direction and then the other.

When the timer goes off, pause. Feel the weight of your body against the floor.

Constraint

- Part of your back should remain on the floor at all times (but how much of your back remains on the floor is open to interpretation).

Key Points

- The limb can glide along the surface or explore the air around you. As you move the limb, can you feel the body responding to the movement?
- Is there anything that felt particularly interesting? If so, what is it?
- Which limb do you prefer to explore with?

Mindful Movement and Play Practice V:
Balance and Integration

For this practice, you will need a ball you are comfortable throwing and catching with one hand and six objects that you can easily pick up with one hand and are approximately the same size.

SEATED FOOT EXPLORATION

Come into a comfortable seated position that allows you to reach your right foot with your hands. This can be done seated in a chair with your right ankle over your left knee, or it can be done on the floor with your ankles crossed in front of you.

Set a timer for two minutes. Pick up your right foot with your hands. Begin moving the foot gently in different directions. You can move the foot so there is movement at the ankle, or you can move the foot so there is movement at the hip. As you move the foot, observe which parts of your leg respond and what it feels like to move slowly and gently. You can even weave the left fingers in between the right toes and move the foot with this hand orientation to see what that feels like.

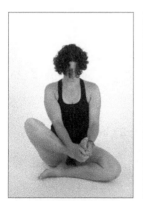 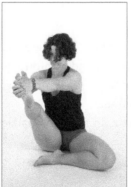 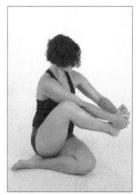

When the timer goes off, pause. Feel your right foot and compare it with your left foot. Do they feel different?

Reset the timer and do the same thing with the left foot.

Constraint

- One hand must be in contact with the foot at all times.

Key Points

- Are you remembering to move gently?
- Which parts of you respond to the movement?
- Which leg feels most responsive to having the foot moved?
- Do you feel more options for moving the foot emerging as time goes on?

USING THE EYES TO MOVE THE HEAD

Set a timer for two minutes. Begin looking around the room. When you see an object or something interesting, let your eyes settle there for a moment, take a couple of breaths, and then allow your eyes to resume scanning the room. Allow your head to respond to the movement of the eyes.

Key Points

- Do you have a preference for where your eyes look?
- Is your head able to respond comfortably to the movement of the eyes? If not, why not?
- Are you able to breathe?
- Do your eyes settle on anything particularly interesting? If so, what is it?

REACHING FROM STANDING

Set up your six objects so they make a geometrical shape in front of you. You can make a six-pointed shape, or a five- or four-pointed shape with one or two of the objects in the middle.

Set a timer for two minutes. Begin standing in the middle of your shape. Lunge a foot forward and use your right hand to touch one of the objects. Return to the standing position. Lunge a foot forward and touch a different object.

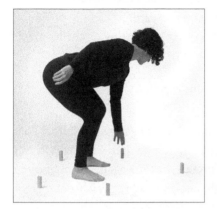
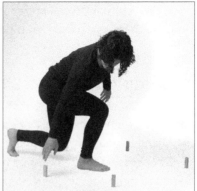

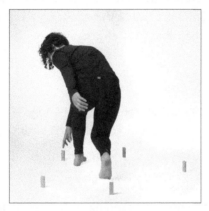

Repeat this, until you have touched all of the objects. Play with using the left and right legs to lunge forward. Change the orientation of your body by facing the shape from a slightly different position or angle. Continue until the timer goes off. Reset the timer and repeat with the other hand.

Constraints

- Touch one object a time.
- The shape should look the same when you finish as it did at the start.

Key Points

- Which hand do you prefer to use to touch the objects?
- Which foot do you prefer to lunge forward?
- Is there a position that is particularly interesting or challenging?

BALANCING WHILE BALL TOSSING

Set a timer for two minutes. Pick up the ball and begin tossing it from your right hand to your left hand, and from your left hand to your right hand.

Once tossing the ball feels comfortable, begin walking as though you were on a tightrope, setting your right heel down directly in front of your left toes and your left heel down directly in front of your right toes, while tossing the ball from one hand to the other. Try to control the ball (and the balance) until the timer goes off.

Constraints

- Keep the ball moving from hand to hand.
- Keep moving one foot directly in front of the other.

Key Points

- Do you find yourself speeding up? What happens if you slow down?
- Do you feel frustrated at all, or do you appreciate the challenge (or maybe it isn't challenging at all)?
- If you find this relatively easy, try doing the same thing on a 2x4, balancing on the 2x4 while tossing the ball from hand to hand. How does that feel?

STANDING TRANSITIONS WITH A BALL

Begin in a standing position. Set a timer for two minutes. Place a ball in the palm of your left hand. While balancing the ball in your hand, practice changing position, balancing on one foot and then the other foot, stepping sideways, turning around in a circle, coming down to one knee and back up again...

Once this becomes comfortable, try standing on one leg and moving the hand away from the body, across the body, overhead, down low, and towards the body. Try not to drop the ball.

Play with different arm positions and moving in different ways until the timer goes off. Reset the timer for two minutes and do the same thing with the ball in the palm of the right hand.

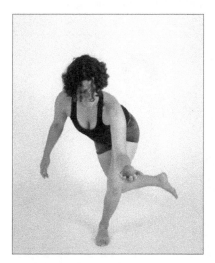 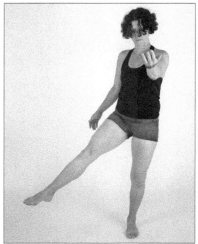

Constraint

- Keep the palm open so the ball is balancing in it the entire time.

Key Points

- Which hand feels more comfortable balancing the ball?
- Do you find yourself moving slowly or quickly? What happens if you move faster? What happens if you move slower?

USING THE BREATH TO MOVE THE HANDS

Come into a comfortable seated position. If you are in a chair, make sure you can feel the feet against the ground and the sitting bones against the chair. If you are on the floor, make sure you can feel the sitting bones supporting you on the ground.

Take your hands to the center of your chest as though you were holding a beach ball. As you inhale, allow your beach ball to get bigger, moving the hands away from each other. As you exhale, allow your beach ball to get smaller, allowing your hands to come towards each other.

Pause for a brief moment, and then begin to exhale, allowing the hands to move up at the same rate of the exhale until they eventually reach the nose. Pause for a moment and begin the inhale again.

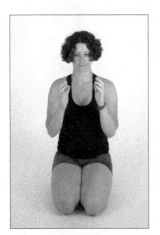 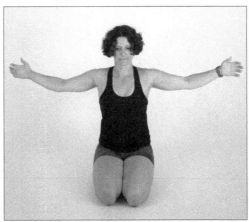

Repeat this pattern for six to eight breath cycles.

When you finish, pause for a moment with your hands by your sides. Feel the sensation of the breath.

Key Points

- How far down do your hands go?
- Can you feel the breath and hands moving at the same rate?
- How quickly do your hands move up?
- Does the tempo change as you repeat the breathing pattern?
- When you finish, are you more or less aware of your breath?

Mindful Movement and Play Practice VI:
Reaching and Grounding

TOP OF THE FOOT TO THE BOTTOM OF THE FOOT

Begin in a standing position with your right foot back and your left foot forward. Roll the right heel off the ground, the right midfoot off the ground, and the bottom of the right toes off the ground. Keep rolling until the top of the foot is on the floor and the bottom of the foot is facing the ceiling.

Reverse the roll, rolling from the top of the foot back to the bottom of the foot. Go back and forth, gently rolling the foot six to eight times. When you finish, pause in standing. Feel the weight of your feet against the floor. Does one foot feel more connected than the other?

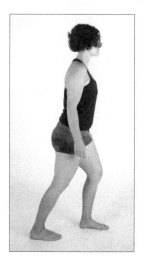 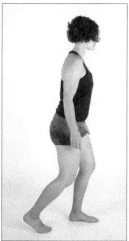 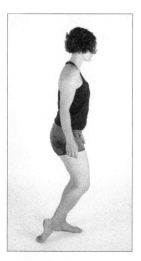

Switch sides, performing the same rolling transition with the left foot.

When you finish, pause with your feet even, breathing gently. Can you feel the weight of your feet against the floor?

Constraints

- Keep the front foot in contact with the floor the entire time.
- Always keep a portion of the back foot in contact with the floor,

even if it's the smallest section of the toes as you roll over the foot during the transition.

Key Points

- Are you breathing?
- Are you allowing the torso to gently shift position, moving forward and back as the foot rolls? Try it both ways: keep the torso completely still and allow it to move. Which way feels more natural?
- Is one side easier than the other?

SEATED REACHING

Set a timer for three minutes. Come into a comfortable seated position on the floor with your legs in whatever orientation you like. If it's uncomfortable to sit on the floor, place a bolster, blanket, or pillow under your pelvis until you are propped up at a height that feel comfortable.

Begin reaching your arms in different positions, towards different places in the room. Every so often, switch the position of your legs and continue reaching. Explore how reaching while the legs are in different positions affects your experience.

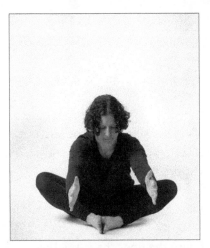 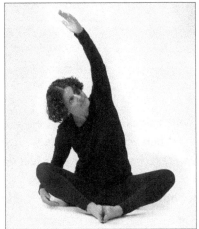

When the timer goes off, pause in a comfortable seated position. Observe your breath for three or four breath cycles.

Constraints

- Keep a portion of the pelvis in contact with the floor the entire time.
- Try to reach towards different places. Even the subtlest shift in reach can make a difference in the experience.

Key Points

- Do the legs respond to the reaching? What happens if you allow the legs to respond to the reaching? What happens if the legs resist the reaching?
- Is there a particular arm or leg position that feels interesting?
- Is there a change in how it feels to be sitting on the floor after the timer goes off?
- Are you choosing to begin and end the exercise in the same position?

SQUAT TRANSITIONS

Set a timer for two minutes. Come into a comfortable squat and stand back up. Change the position of the feet or arms and squat again. Continue with this, squatting a little bit differently each time, until the timer goes off.

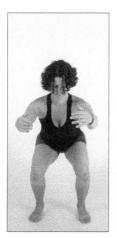 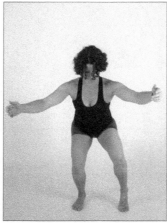 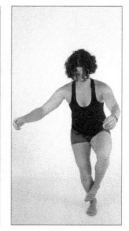

Constraints

- There is no depth limit. Just squat to a comfortable place you know you can stand up from.
- One foot must be in contact with the floor at all times (the emphasis isn't on jumping squats).

Key Points

- What position do you find most interesting for your feet?
- What position do you find most interesting for your arms?
- Is there a position that is particularly challenging for you? Why is it challenging?

ROLLING ON THE FLOOR

Set a timer for three minutes. Lie on your back with your legs long and your arms long by your side.

Explore the space around you with your left hand. As you explore the space, can you begin to figure out how you could use your left arm and hand to roll over onto your right side? Try not to force anything, just see what options come up.

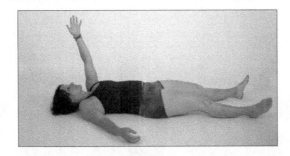

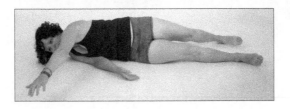

After spending some time with that, switch to your right hand and arm, then to your right leg, and finally to your left leg.

When the timer goes off, rest on your back for three or four breaths, observing the contact you make with the floor.

Constraints

- Avoid using extra effort (see how easily you can find ways to roll).
- Try to lead with one limb at a time.
- The limb can come off the floor or stay on the floor.

Key Points

- Can you feel your torso responding to the exploration of the arm or leg?
- Is it easier to lead with the arm or leg?
- Are you finding ways to transition onto your side?
- Are you able to find ways that feel easy? Or is it difficult to not over-effort the movement?

As you can see, there are many ways to approach short practices that create mindfulness through focused attention, breathing, grounding, and centering. The key points are guides for self-reflection and assist with listening. It can be argued that several other practices, such as parkour, circus arts, martial arts, and dance, are all mindful movement practices. People who don't like traditional fitness settings can often find a practice that resonates by exploring more alternative physical practices.

The goal of using physical movement in enhancing mental well-being shouldn't be to force people to do things they dislike. Rather, exploring different ways of moving the body in a way that feels interesting and invites curiosity increases the likelihood that the individual will continue and make movement a lifelong habit.

One of the many roles of the practitioner is to tap into the interests of the student. I have a client who is about to turn 80. She loves ball games (and she is really good at them). As a result, I include play activities that involve tossing balls in a variety of ways. The enjoyment she gets from the ball work makes the strength work more palatable (and the physical and mental benefits she has experienced because she feels stronger have reinforced the importance of the strength work).

Play doesn't have to be lost just because adulthood is reached. Letting go of rigid instructions and encouraging exploration is a way to introduce play back into a person's life. Play has far-reaching implications related to learning, creativity, and mental function; it's worth inviting it into the movement practice regularly.

References

Darling-Hammond L., Flook L., Cook-Harvey C., Barron B., & Osher D. (2020). Implications for educational practice of the science of learning and development. Applied Developmental Science, 24(2), 97-140.

Guitard P., Ferland F., Dutil E. (2005). Toward a better understanding of playfulness in adults. OTJR: Occupation, Participation, and Health, 25(1), 9-22.

Kwakkel G., Veerbeek J.M., van Wegen E.E.H., & Wolf S.L. (2015). Constraint-induced movement therapy after stroke. Lancet Neurology, 14(2), 224-234.

Rohde M., Narioka K., Steil J.J., Klein L.K., & Ernst M.O. (2019). Goal related feedback guides motor exploration and redundancy resolution in human motor skill acquisition. PLOS Computer Biology, 15(3), 1-27.

Russ S.W., & Wallace C.E. (2013). Pretend play and creative processes. American Journal of Play, 6(1), 136-148.

Sullivan K.J., Kantak S.S., & Burtner P.A. (2008). Motor learning in children: Feedback effects on skill acquisition. Physical Therapy, 88(6), 720-732.

Wilson R.C., Shenhav A., Straccia M., & Cohen J.D. (2019). The eighty-five percent rule for optimal learning. Nature Communications, 10, 4646.

Zeng N., Ayyub M., Sun H., Wen X., Xiang P., & Gao Z. (2017). Effects of physical activity on motor skills and cognitive development in early childhood: A systematic review. Biomed Research International, 2017, 2760716.

Zosh J.M., Hirsh-Pasek K., Hopkins E.J., Jensen H., et al. (2018). Accessing the inaccessible: Redefining play as a spectrum. Frontiers in Psychology, 9, 124.

CHAPTER 10

Putting It All Together

Now that you understand how different aspects of movement, specifically endurance, strength, mobility, and mindful movement, impact mental health and well-being, you may be wondering how it can all be incorporated into a session. The goal isn't for you to throw out what you have been teaching and what you already know; rather, the goal behind the words and science on these pages is to deepen your knowledge about how movement can impact the entire person. This, in turn, can help you provide guidance, design workshops and retreats, and facilitate what you decide to include with clients, depending on their individual tendencies. For instance, I don't come from a dance background; however, I have taken several workshops based on dance principles and I have learned how to incorporate some of those principles into sessions and courses, specifically improvisational drills and non-contact partner drills. These drills require active listening and focused attention and don't have a goal-specific outcome, which makes them a great choice when I am working with clients who would benefit mentally and physically from exploring movement in that way.

If you are a Pilates instructor, be a Pilates instructor; if you are a yoga teacher, be a yoga teacher; and if you are a strength and conditioning coach, be a strength and conditioning coach, but understand how other components of movement and fitness fit in to your client's psychological health. The rest of this chapter is devoted to designing movement-based training and the evidence behind program design. Some of the evidence is sparse, and not all of the recommendations will apply to whatever it is you teach, but it's worth exploring and may give you insights or ideas for clients who are less responsive or more difficult to work with. To begin, let's explore the initial aspect of a session: the warm-up.

Movement Warm-Up

Most systems have some variation of a warm-up. It's traditionally meant to increase blood flow, prep the neuromuscular system for more complex activity, and transition the client into physical activity. In baseball players, high-load dynamic warm-ups increase power and strength performance (both of which are beneficial while playing baseball). It has been found that static stretching, on the other hand, doesn't affect power outcomes at all, and data showed hanging out with a heat or ice pack before playing to be mostly ineffective (McCrary *et al.*, 2015).

When soccer players used a dynamic warm-up that included dynamic stretching and short sprints, their sprinting speed improved while they were playing. When another group of soccer players used things like core stability, balance, muscle activation, strength/plyometric exercises, and partner running drills to warm up, their sprinting speed during play didn't improve. This suggests that if the goal is to warm up for soccer, you should probably do things that resemble playing soccer (Ayala *et al.*, 2017). And as you will see in a minute, if the goal is to warm up for a specific movement skill, you should probably do things in your warm-up that resemble the actual skill.

What if the goal is to reduce injury risk? While there is no way to prevent all injuries, research does suggest that targeted neuromuscular warm-ups may be an effective way to reduce injuries (at least in the lower body) (Herman *et al.*, 2012).

This should make sense. If you have been sitting at a desk for three hours and then get up and begin lifting weights on your lunch break, your entire system has to reroute from expending little physical energy to moving vigorously. Spending three to five minutes reconnecting your brain to your body through targeted neuromuscular exercises gets the nervous system primed for more complex movements; it also shifts blood flow out to the extremities and changes how you are feeling—it's not unusual for people who don't feel like exercising to comment five to ten minutes later, "I feel so much better." This is because of the neurotransmitters (specifically dopamine and serotonin) that flood your system when you move. This makes you feel more energetic and alert and might even make the world seem like a better place (Basso & Suzuki, 2017).

Finally, a warm-up that includes neuromuscular exercises may be a way to improve the effectiveness of a targeted strength-based program. When adults with a meniscus tear participated in an exercise program that comprised five minutes on a stationary bike, eight neuromuscular exercises that targeted improving awareness and motor control in the lower leg, and four leg-strengthening exercises, knee pain decreased. In fact, six months after completing the exercise intervention, none of the participants had opted or were waiting for knee surgery (Skou & Thorlund, 2018).

What does all of this tell us about how warm-ups can be used in a session that is focusing on a holistic approach? The people in these studies were young, some were not even adults, and chances are high that you work with a variety of ages (including people in their 40s and older). However, designing an effective warm-up for your client isn't all that different from designing an effective warm-up for an athlete or improving sensorimotor control for someone with knee pain. The warm-up should improve body awareness and connection to the areas that are going to be emphasized or used throughout the session. The motor patterns should be relevant to the exercises you are going to highlight during your session. If there is an element of grounding or centering, the warm-up exercises can also be an opportunity to focus.

Let's say your last client of the day is a 55-year-old patent lawyer named Ben who spends his day reading contracts and helping people protect their intellectual property. He spends most of the day at his desk, though he does get up and move around at lunch time if he doesn't have any conference calls or meetings. He is prone to work-induced anxiety, has the occasional bout of back pain, and gets tension headaches. He also runs six miles five days a week to stay in shape. What should his warm-up focus on?

There are no wrong answers, and I think we can agree that any movement will benefit him, given that he spends most of his day in one position. Incorporating dynamic mobility that targets his spine, wrists, ankles, feet, shoulders, and neck will serve as a reminder that: a) all of these areas are capable of moving multiple ways and b) there is a body connected to his well-exercised brain.

How you structure the warm-up can look a lot of different ways. When I work with people who don't use their bodies regularly through-out the day, I tend to start on the ground so they can begin re-establishing a connection to their physical location in space.

From there, I gradually work up to a standing position, transitioning from more neuromuscular/awareness work to more strength-based work. In my experience, people with intellectually demanding jobs who don't move much during their workday think less about their bodies during the day than the yoga teacher who teaches 26 classes a week. As a result, I prioritize giving them time to feel different parts of their physical structure. This makes it easier for them to implement different instructions. If they haven't thought about their feet for three days and I direct awareness to the feet, it takes the brain a minute to connect my words with the body part. If they have already felt their feet during the warm-up, it's much easier and faster to grasp the experience of using their feet. This translates into them feeling good during their movement session and enhances their overall experience.

Before I move on, I should note that neuromuscular/sensorimotor training is simply movement with an awareness of how the movement is being performed. It can feel like a strength exercise, like a mobility exercise, or like it's both strengthening and mobilizing. These types of exercises may use bands or light resistance to improve kinesthetic awareness, reduce degrees of freedom, or provide general tactile feedback, but the emphasis is on control and feeling rather than improving strength, power, or endurance. Because the warm-up exercises enhance the overall practice, I often use this time to start directing attention to the area I want to emphasize throughout the session. If I want the client to feel their ribs, I will use exercises that mobilize the rib cage and begin directing attention to the ribs in various positions. The warm-up becomes an introduction to the session as a whole, allowing the client to focus attention and begin generating curiosity.

The duration of the warm-up depends on the length of the session. For a 55-minute session, I usually design the warm-up to last 5–12 minutes. Neuromuscular and dynamic mobility exercises can also be used as fillers between strength-based exercises, so don't worry if you don't get to all of the awareness exercises during the first portion of the session. You can always work them in later.

What If You Are Doing a Restorative-Based Session?

Incorporating a warm-up as a way to focus attention and create a sense of grounding and centering is useful in restorative-based sessions. It may be done using the floor as a way to facilitate a mind/body connection using supine or seated movement and eventually segueing into more complex motor patterns with an emphasis on efficiency.

Complex rolling patterns on the floor, for instance, can be quite restorative but require an element of skill. Once people learn how to do them, they can be a great warm-up, but they can also be built up to during a session and positioned after things like gentle mobility work and rocking patterns have been introduced.

Think of the warm-up as a reintroduction to the body. Take our hypothetical client, Ben. Movements that mobilize the spine, hips, and wrists and remind him that there is more to him than his cognitive self will make him feel better physically and mentally. This primes the entire system for more challenging movements.

After the Warm-Up: A Strength-Based Session

What do you do after you have warmed up? You move the client into the working part of the session. This might mean the movements that require the most focus (because that certainly falls under the category of work) or it might mean the movements that are hard for the client. I find that getting the hardest things out of the way early makes the rest of the session more enjoyable. When people are working on building strength, the strength-building part of the session often feels the most like work.

What is required to build strength? You learned in Chapter 3 that building strength requires a loading of the tissues through progressive overload, but how do you program strength training into a session in a way that maximizes effectiveness?

A Quick Overview of Terms

"Repetition" (or rep) refers to the number of times you do the same movement pattern, so if I lift a dumbbell up and down ten times, I have done ten repetitions.

"Set" refers to how many groups of reps you perform. If I lift my dumbbell up and down ten times, rest, and then lift it up and down ten more times, I have done two sets of ten dumbbell lifts. If I do ten push-ups, hang on the monkey bars for ten seconds, and repeat this sequence four times, I have performed four sets of ten reps of push-ups and four sets of one ten-second monkey-bar hang.

"1RM" refers to your one-repetition maximum. If I know I can lift 225 pounds once using a deadlift pattern, I know that my 1RM for the deadlift is 225. If I want to perform the deadlift using a set/rep scheme and I want the weight to be moderate so I can lift it eight to ten times, I will figure out what 60 percent of my 1RM is (135 pounds), and I will use that weight to perform my sets and reps. Most people don't know what their 1RM is, and it's not really worth figuring it out unless someone specifically wants to improve their 1RM (and if that's the case, you should refer them to someone who specializes in that type of strength and conditioning). A better indicator for the general person who wants to get stronger is gauging intensity. Is the person able to lift the weight comfortably eight to ten times? If it feels relatively light after the tenth repetition, it's probably not heavy enough to elicit a strengthening response. If the person begins to struggle with the weight after five repetitions, it's an appropriate weight for working on power but may be heavy for working on strength.

What Is the Difference between Strength and Power?

Strength is the ability to exert force. The goal of improving squat strength requires the neuromuscular system to have the ability to gradually improve its tolerance of higher amounts of load while the body is moving through a squatting pattern. One definition of strength says that strength is the ability to maximally generate force at a specific velocity (Everett, 1993). Using the squat as an example, the person who can squat slowly under load is building a different type of strength than the person who uses the squat as a way to generate force for jumping. Both require strength, but moving slowly isn't the same as moving fast and moving fast isn't the same as moving slowly.

Power is the ability to generate force in the shortest amount of time. When the person squats slowly under load, it takes a long time to move through the repetition. This uses less power than when the person squats down and then explodes up.

Power is also used if you squat down without weight and then explode up, jump off the floor, and then land back in a squat. The jump squat requires more explosiveness than the slow, controlled squat that is emphasizing strength. Both will make you stronger, just in different ways.

Power and strength both decrease with age, and power appears to decrease faster than muscle strength. However, research suggests that traditional strength training is as effective as power training for improving maximal strength, muscle power, and lower-limb functional performance in elderly women (Tiggemann *et al.*, 2016). This is great news because it means if someone despises jumping for whatever reason, they can still get strong and improve their ability to generate power regardless of their age. Conversely, if someone loves jumping and power-based movements, they can use them to improve strength and function.

Determining how many sets and reps to perform should be based on the individual's current training status. Let's take Ben, the patent lawyer we met earlier in the chapter. He hasn't done any strength training in 20 years (running falls into the category of endurance training). Not only would he benefit from learning new positions and movements required to perform the movement patterns associated with strength training, he also needs to build up a solid foundation and understanding of how his body moves to support the new stress of strength training.

Research suggests that using light loads of 45–50 percent of the 1RM may be enough to increase dynamic muscular strength (Kraemer & Ratamess, 2004). This means that using a load that feels comfortable is a good starting place for new exercisers. They can also just use body weight initially or use light weights to give kinesthetic feedback about position. The benefit of this strategy is that if you teach people how to perform the movements in a situation that feels safe, they will be able to groove the movement pattern so it feels comfortable and consistent. This translates to movement patterns that perform well under load and gives the client the ability to self-correct. If Ben can feel whether his front hip rotates back in a staggered stance position, that means he will feel when it doesn't rotate back when he is doing a split-stance deadlift.

Using light loads will also give Ben a chance to try different things and feel what works for his body without being worried he might hurt himself. It's a lot easier to adjust the feet to see what feels most support-ive when you are lifting a weight you can move ten times than it is to do so when you are using a weight you can only lift four times.

After a month, Ben will begin feeling more capable and confident in his abilities. This means he will feel more confident to use heavier loads and perform more repetitions. I often start people with four or five repetitions of new exercises with a light load. This gives them an opportunity to go slowly, make errors with low risk of injury, and begin learning the components of the movement that are necessary to success-fully complete the skill in an efficient way. It also reduces the amount of soreness associated with new exercise programs and gives the entire neuromuscular system a chance to adapt to the new activity.

Ben will quickly adapt to the new stimulus, both neurologically and physiologically. As this happens, he can be challenged with higher load and more volume. Volume refers to the total amount of work performed in a single session. Once Ben has been strength training for several months, if he wants to continue increasing muscular hypertrophy, he will need to use heavy loads (greater than 80–85 percent 1RM). Research suggests that the initial increases in strength that happen when someone begins strength training are because of neural adaptations (Jenkins *et al.*, 2017). Basically, your CNS figures out that in order to lift something heavy off the floor, it needs to recruit more motor units and have them work together in a synchronous way (the nervous system is incredibly smart when it comes to these sorts of things). Once that happens, the muscles adapt by getting bigger.

If someone has been strength training for a long time, the only way to jumpstart the neural adaptations is by using heavy loads. This means that if you want to become more efficient at deadlifting, an effective way to do this is to use heavier weights.

Most people don't need to continually get stronger. They need to attain a base level of strength that makes everyday life feel easy and makes them feel like they aren't breakable, and then they need to use that strength a lot of different ways. In order to begin developing musculoskeletal strength, clients need to be exposed to more than one set per exercise. This means that when Ben starts out using light loads, he will need to do more than one set to get stronger. However, how much more than one set is required is up for debate (Ralston *et al.*, 2017). Using a graded-exposure approach (starting with two sets, gradually working up to three sets, and maybe eventually working up to four sets) will support the client's continued ability to adapt to the workload and get more efficient. Almost everyone notices how much easier an exercise is the second time through, regardless of whether it's strength, balance, or mobility. This is likely due to the learning effect that accompanies random-order practice. If I do a handstand, do a set of pull-ups, and then do another handstand, my handstands will probably get better faster than if I do a handstand, rest, and do another handstand. If I really wanted to improve my handstands, I would do handstands randomly throughout the day, but again, that isn't the goal for most people. You can use the concept of random-order practice by programming things like supersets (performing two exercises, one right after another, with minimal rest), interval training, or circuits with your clients (Getchell et al., 2018).

There are several limitations that exist in the strength-training research on finding the perfect number of sets. Sample sizes are usually small, which makes it difficult to generalize about whether the results will work for most people. Something else to consider is that women often respond differently to the training protocols than men. This is probably due to a number of factors, including genetics, hormonal factors, age, and current stress level. Of course, these differences exist between everyone, but the biological differences between a man and a woman are different to those between two men or two women (Ralston et al., 2017).

What you can take away from this is no two people are alike. If you are programming strength training into your work with clients, pay attention to how they respond and how they feel. That is a good way to gauge what you need to tinker with and which variables (like volume) you need to change.

Back to the original point: what should a strength-training protocol look like for someone who is brand new to strength work and would benefit from increasing their general strength and stability? Let's look at two individuals, a yoga teacher with benign JHS named Mary and a nurse who isn't hypermobile but has bouts of neck pain named Janice.

Mary and Janice are both active 43-year-olds. Mary teaches 12 yoga classes a week and maintains a yoga practice. She feels like her sacroiliac (SI) joint slips, and she has been noticing a general ache throughout her low back and pelvis. She is worried something may be wrong structurally, and she feels general anxiety about her ability to continue teaching.

Janice hikes regularly and is on her feet all day at work. She experiences high levels of work stress and is worried about changes her department is making and the impact those changes will have on her. Her dad passed away three years ago; her mom still lives by herself but is having trouble keeping the house clean, and Janice worries her mom may be exhibiting signs of forgetfulness. Janice's neck pain has been intermittent over the years but it seems to be happening more frequently. She had imaging done, but the doctor told her she didn't have any structural issues in her cervical spine.

Mary needs general strength that is built slowly using graded exposure to load. Because she is hypermobile, she will feel safest with fewer degrees of freedom. This means her program should use positions that utilize lots of sensory feedback and externally focused instructions. Her program should focus on creating a general sense of stability through thoughtful, progressive loads. Initially, a low-volume scheme should be used that emphasizes the sensation of work and builds coordination and neuromuscular efficiency in positions like the squat, hip hinge, upper body pressing, and pulling.

Mary is also extremely body aware, so after four to six weeks, she will likely begin to feel stronger and more confident. As this happens, movements can become slightly more complex and volume can increase slightly. If you do too much too soon with Mary, not only will she feel sore, but she may also feel injured or worried about the risk of injury. With slow, gradual exposure Mary will thrive.

Janice, though she is active, is less body aware and not as comfortable on the floor. Janice also isn't very flexible; the idea of bending over to touch her toes makes Janice grimace. Janice will benefit from strength moves that also increase her mobility, with an emphasis on staying connected to her center of mass (Janice, like many people with neck pain, visibly lifts her head and chest away from the rest of her torso. This not only alters her breathing pattern and makes her neck feel tight, but it also decreases her ability to feel both centered and grounded.)

Janice also needs gradual exposure to volume, but she will benefit from using a more dynamic approach to positions rather than an isometric approach. Load only needs to be used at first to help Janice feel positions and decrease degrees of freedom when necessary (this is in contrast to Mary, who will initially benefit from some sort of sensory feedback in almost every position). Janice will make improvements rapidly, and after about four weeks, the volume can begin to increase.

Both can use a similar set/rep scheme at a manageable intensity. If any of the positions used are new or unfamiliar, they may initially feel intense muscular work that will lessen with repeated exposure to the position. It would be good to start with two or three sets of 10–30-second isometric holds for Mary and two or three sets of four to six reps for Janice.

In both cases, once the initial exposure to the new movements feels safe and manageable, they will learn to trust that they are strong and they can withstand the work. This will increase their work tolerance, resulting in strength gains and feelings of confidence and capability.

Skills and Play

Here is an unscientific view of programming that I utilize all of the time: strength training feels like work, so I place it earlier in a session while people have the energy and motivation to deal with doing something that is physically challenging. I usually program skill work and play after strength work because it's fun and generally more interesting.

There is one caveat: if you are doing a heavy lifting session with a client, they may experience neuromuscular fatigue, which could impact their capacity for coordinated movement. For instance, if you program a lot of overhead pressing movements during the strength portion and move into handstand training for the skill work, the handstand work may be shorter than you originally intended. To be perfectly honest, the only person I have working on handstands right now is me, and if I want a rewarding handstand practice, I don't do it on days I am doing a lot of overhead pressing. *Most* people need general strength and their skill- and play-based work is less acrobatic. Skill and play work can include things like walking across a 2x4 in a variety of ways or balancing on a rail, ground work that is playful, like rolls, or games with a ball.

Certain movements, like crawling, are both strength building and potentially more playful in nature. Which category movements fall into depends on the client: their current level of endurance and strength, their personal preferences, and what they do outside of their time with you can all impact their view of a specific movement. Some of my clients find crawling interesting and enjoy interspersing it with an element of play because they have already built up the endurance needed to crawl for a long period of time; others groan when I ask them to come into the starting position for a crawl because they find it hard.

I also find the period after strength training a great time to teach a new variation of a body-weight movement or skill. There is a repetitiveness to strength training that allows people to count reps and not focus so much on coordinating how the right arm moves with the right leg that I find translates well into more focused learning later. Plus, there is the general sense of muscular effort which accompanies weightlifting that leads to improvements in interoception, proprioception, and general kinesthetic awareness; this increased body sense seems to make it easier for people to feel what they are doing as they navigate their bodies in new ways.

Many traditional strength-based exercises can be very grounding and centering, depending on how they're taught. For instance, in a movement like a goblet squat, holding a weight in the middle of the chest causes you to orient around the weight. This makes it easier to feel centered, which translates well to skills that require an element of balance.

The feet are used during a goblet squat as reference points and to generate force. Depending on how you instruct the movement and where you ask the client to focus their attention, the feet and their contact with the floor can be a focal point for grounding that carries over into other movements.

Skill and play work can be programmed in a few different ways. You can use a timer, which gives people the space to work on the task as much or as little as they want until the timer goes off. If you are using partner-based work, a timer tends to work well and allows the partners to focus on the task.

You can also superset skill and play work with another exercise using something similar to a set/rep scheme. I often do this with balance work because people will fixate and want to try repeatedly until they get it; what they don't realize is that stepping away, doing something else, and then returning to the balance task often makes them more successful. If they know that they will have an opportunity to return to the balance challenge, they can be less concerned if they don't "get" it the first time.

One of the things I find interesting about this approach is that knowing there is something potentially fun or rewarding happening later appears to make the strength work more digestible. (Not that lifting heavy things isn't rewarding; it is. But there is something incredibly inspiring about watching people embody a movement skill that they have been working towards for a long time. The feeling of body control people experience when they realize that they are athletic and coordinated is a pleasure to witness.) Even when a play task is woven into a more challenging strength-based skill like active hanging variations or single-leg squat variations, the creativity and focused attention required during play-based tasks often supersede the potential sensation of work.

And this, from a psychological point of view, makes sense. People are most likely to experience a state of flow when there is an element of challenge or work. It's not that work is pleasurable exactly, just like writing over 80,000 words on the effects of exercise on mental health isn't exactly fun, but the focus required to navigate how to achieve the goal, whether it's to not drop the ball or to disseminate information in a way that is relatable, is challenging enough to drown out the endless chatter of the monkey mind, focus attention, and optimize awareness (Tozman *et al.*, 2017).

The Cool-Down

After the strength has been built, games have been played, and attention has been focused, it's time to return to more centering and grounding work. Again, what counts as a cool-down is client dependent, but I like to end with smaller movements in a position that is grounding, whether that's seated or in a comfortable, non-threatening position on the floor. Sometimes I conclude with gentle movements that center the person (rocking side to side or forward and back), and sometimes I bring the focus to the breath. This not only serves to downregulate the SNS, but it also gives me an opportunity to see how the person responded to the session. When people initially lie down on the floor at the beginning of a session, it's not uncommon to see a lack of settling, which appears as ribs that are lifted from the floor, a pelvis that is tipped one way, or a shoulder that's lifting up and away from the ground. A well-structured movement practice will bring a person back into a place that feels more balanced, both physically and emotionally.

What about a Mindful Movement or Restorative Session?

Not everyone needs strength-based work. If someone regularly strength trains and is still experiencing anxiety or moments of panic, they may need more balance between the PSNS and SNS. A program that takes a more restorative approach will provide a high amount of benefit. Many of the aspects will look the same—there will still be a warm-up to introduce awareness in the body, which will likely be ground based, followed by subtle work on whatever you want to emphasize, maybe the foot, hand, pelvis, shoulder blades... After the warm-up is a great time to tap into the area you want to emphasize and the surrounding areas.

Once that's finished, strength is replaced by thoughtful movement that is grounding and centering, including balance work and floor work. This segues into more dynamic exposure to the area using play-based tasks (the dance world is a great source for ideas). Eventually, the exploration winds down and the person is placed in a position that is centering and grounding, using the breath or open monitoring to end.

Putting It All Together

You can probably tell that many of these session sections bleed into one another. While it's difficult to place a singular task in just one category, it is possible to design a movement practice that hits all of the categories in a relatively seamless way.

Below are sample programs for the people discussed throughout the chapter. Before you read through my examples, take the time to write out your own strength-based sample programs for these individuals.

The goal isn't to compare your sample program with mine and decide which is right; it's simply to observe how many ways there are to approach the same person. The ideas I present below are based on my training and experience. Your programs will be based on your training and experience. Neither is better than the other, and, hopefully, if you noticed there were concepts you were less familiar with as you went through these chapters, your curiosity was piqued. What makes a great practitioner is the desire to continue learning, a personal movement practice that is robust, the desire to be exposed to a wide variety of techniques and modalities, and, of course, the ability to listen.

Sample practices

Ben (Lawyer, Runs Regularly, Prone to Anxiety)

WARM-UP

Mobility Work

1. Scapular elevation and depression, open chain.
2. Open-chain scapular retraction and protraction and closed-chain scapular protraction and retraction.
3. Spinal mobility (cat/cow with the arms and legs in different positions).

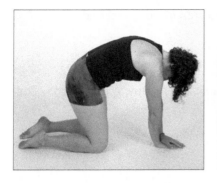 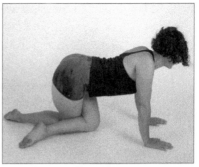

4. Ankle rolls, open chain.
5. Heel raises with the emphasis on feeling the balls of the feet.

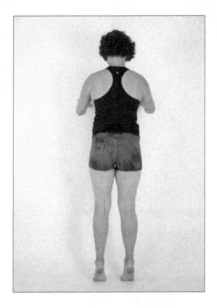

6. Down dog transition to squat.

STRENGTH WORK
Circuit I (3 Sets)

1. Loaded lunge variations (performed slowly with the emphasis on instructing the feet and the relationship to the pelvis): 8 repetitions per side.
2. Push-ups (hands in different positions): 10 repetitions.

3. Hanging (load the arms as tolerated): 10–30 seconds.

Circuit II (3 Sets)

1. Goblet squats (instruct the feet and go slowly, pause at the bottom): 10 repetitions.

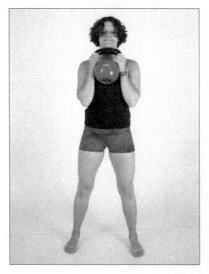 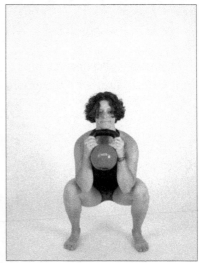

2. Farmer's carries: 2 laps of 15 feet.
3. Staggered stance rows (pay attention to the pelvis and torso position): 8 per side.

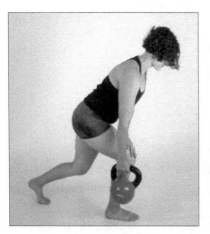 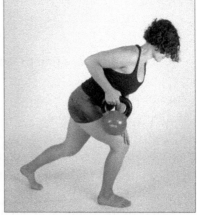

Circuit III (3 Sets)

1. Kickstand deadlifts (instruct the feet and pelvis): 6 per side.
2. Crawling around obstacles: 2 laps of 15 feet.
3. Tall kneeling lean back (pay attention to the torso position). Add in spinal mobility work if applicable (when Ben feels stiff through his neck and shoulders): 6 repetitions.

Circuit IV (3 Sets)

1. Balance: 2x4 walk and touch (touch objects on the ground while moving across the 2x4): 2 laps of 16 feet.

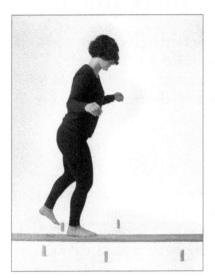 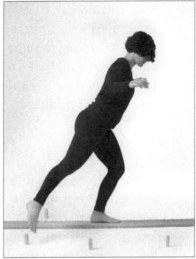

2. Teacups, variation one: 45 seconds per side.
3. Tripod get-up: 6 per side.

COOL-DOWN

1. Gentle arm movement, shoulder movement, and neck movement.
2. Breathing in a comfortable position.

Mary (Hypermobile Yoga Teacher)

WARM-UP

1. Dying bug stability drills (use props).
2. Single-leg bridging with the emphasis on hip extension (not lumbar extension), and pelvis position.
3. Prone swimmers (with the emphasis on reaching and maintaining torso position).

CIRCUIT I (3 SETS)

1. Tall kneeling banded pull-apart (with the emphasis on maintaining rib position and feeling work in the back of the shoulder): 6-10 repetitions.
2. Quadruped rows (with the emphasis on keeping the torso and pelvis still during rowing action): 6–8 per side.
3. Tall half-kneeling back-knee lifts using a plyo box for the hands to maintain the rib position (with the emphasis on the pelvis position): 2–4 per side.

CIRCUIT II (3 SETS)

1. Suitcase lowers (with the emphasis on the torso and pelvis position, as well as instructing for grip): 4–6 repetitions.
2. Elevated push-ups on a plyo box (with the emphasis on slowly lowering down and maintaining the torso position throughout the movement—use additional props, like a yoga block between the thighs or feet, as needed): 8–10 repetitions.
3. Goblet squats: 6–18 repetitions.

CIRCUIT III (3 SETS)

1. Skater squat knee tap down to yoga block (feel the foot connection; the front heel can lift in the bottom position): 4–6 per side.

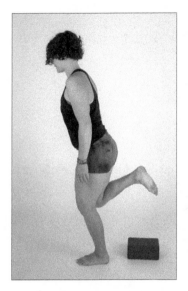 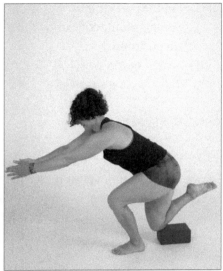

2. Tall kneeling position lat pull-down: 6–8 repetitions.
3. Balance: Step to 2x4, tripod leg through: 2–4 per side.

CIRCUIT IV (3 SETS)

1. Bottoms-up half-kneeling kettlebell external rotation (hand on the wall to maintain torso position): 4–6 per side.
2. Step-up variation: 4–6 per side.
3. Prone hip flexion (feet on towel, maintain torso position): 4–6 repetitions.

COOL-DOWN

1. Breathing, focus on the rib position with a long exhale (maybe use child's pose/rounded back position).
2. Supine breathing, block between the feet, long exhale, feel the ribs and pelvic floor working together.

Janice (Nurse, Not Very Flexible, Neck Pain, Anxious)
WARM-UP

1. Supine neck nods.

2. Supine pelvic tilts.
3. Supine shoulder flexion with exhale (with the emphasis on the rib position).
4. Seated 90/90 switches.
5. Tall kneeling sit backs.

CIRCUIT I (3 SETS)

1. Get up from the floor, get down to the floor (do it differently each time): set a timer for 60 seconds.
2. Plank walk-outs: 6–8 repetitions.
3. Plank rotate to side plank: 4–6 per side.

CIRCUIT II (3 SETS)

1. Multi-planar lunge: 6–8 per side.
2. Prone seated hip bridge to elevated long sit (hands elevated on parallettes bars or yoga blocks): 4–6 repetitions.
3. Farmer's carries across 2x4: 2 laps.

CIRCUIT III (3 SETS)

1. Kettlebell clean to squat: 6–8 repetitions.
2. Multi-planar single-leg reach (touching an object, with the foot or hand): 30–45 seconds per leg.
3. Straight arm hang (active to passive): 10–30 seconds.

CIRCUIT IV (3 SETS)

1. Figure-four rock backs: 4–6 per side.
2. Kneeling get-ups (modified): 4–6 per side.
3. Knee hand hip roll. (See if these can flow together by the last round): 2–4 per side.

COOL-DOWN

1. Seated positions (long sit, butterfly, cross-legged). Hold each new position for 30 seconds before moving on to the next position. Cycle through twice.
2. Cat/cow.
3. End in child's pose for breathing.

References

Ayala F., Calderon-Lopez A., Delgado-Gosalbez J.C., Parra-Sanchez S., *et al.* (2017). Acute effects of three neuromuscular warm-up strategies on several physical performance measures in football players. PLOS ONE, 12(1), 1-17.

Basso J.C., & Suzuki W.A. (2017). The effects of acute exercise on mood, cognition, neurophysiology, and neurochemical pathways: A review. Brain Plasticity, 2(2), 127-152.

Everett H. (1993). Strength and power: A definition of terms. National Strength and Conditioning Association Journal, 15(6), 18-21.

Getchell N., Schilder A., Wusch E., & Trask A. (2018). Chapter 86: A Random Practice Schedule Provides Better Retention and Transfer Than Blocked When Learning Computer Mazes: Preliminary Results, 303-304. In: Neuroergonomics: The Brain at Work and in Everyday Life. Cambridge, MA: Elsevier.

Herman K., Barton C., Malliaras P., & Morrissey D. (2012). The effectiveness of neuromuscular warm-up strategies, that require no additional equipment, for preventing lower limb injuries during sports participation: A systematic review. BMC Medicine, 10, 75.

Jenkins N.D.M., Miramoni A.A., Hill E.C., Smith C.M., *et al.* (2017). Greater neural adaptations following high- vs. low-load resistance training. Frontiers in Physiology, 8, 331.

Kraemer W.J., & Ratamess N.A. (2004). Fundamentals of resistance progression and exercise. Medicine & Science in Sports & Exercise, 36(4), 674-686.

McCrary J.M., Ackermann B.J., & Halaki M. (2015). A systematic review of the effects of upper body warm-up on performance and injury. British Journal of Sports Medicine, 49(14), 935-942.

Ralston G.W., Kilgore L., Wyatt F.B., & Baker J.S. (2017). The effect of weekly set volume on strength gain: A meta-analysis. Sports Medicine, 47, 2585-2601.

Skou S.T., & Thorlund J.B. (2018). A 12-week supervised exercise therapy program for young adults with a meniscal tear: Program development and feasibility study. Journal of Bodywork and Movement Therapies, 22(3), 786-791.

Tiggemann C.L., Dias C.P., Radaelli R., Massa J.C., *et al.* (2016). Effect of traditional resistance and power training using rated perceived exertion for enhancement of muscle strength, power, and functional performance. Age, 38(2), 42.

Tozman T., Zhang Y.Y., & Vollmeyer R. (2017). Inverted u-shaped function between flow and cortisol release during chess play. Journal of Happiness Studies: An Interdisciplinary Forum on Subjective Well-Being, 18(1), 247-268.

Conclusion

While I discussed mood disorders and the research surrounding anxiety, depression, and post-traumatic stress, the benefits of movement extend beyond those three conditions. Exercise has been implicated as a positive intervention for a number of other neurological conditions that can affect mental health, including attention deficit disorder (Mehren *et al.*, 2020), autism spectrum disorder (Ferreira *et al.*, 2019), and schizophrenia (Girdler *et al.*, 2019).

Hopefully, the potential mechanisms behind the benefits of movement and exercise make sense—exercise literally changes your brain. It is, of course, not a panacea for poor mental health, which is multi-faceted, but it is an important piece of the puzzle, and if people with mental health conditions seek the expertise of a movement professional, there is suddenly more at play than just the exercise component. The interaction between two human beings can impact a person's experience in a profound way.

While Part II of this book was devoted to movement, exercise, and ideas for exploring concepts related to mobility, improving body awareness, play, and strength, my hope is that you can see the possibilities for movement interventions are, actually, endless. I discussed a variety of modalities but not all modalities—the benefits to activities like martial arts, circus arts, and dance can also be worth pursuing if more common modalities don't seem to be resonating. One way a practitioner can support a person's mental health and well-being is to support the journey to finding an activity that facilitates a sense of accomplishment and strength in the student or client.

The more open-minded you are as a practitioner, the easier it is to create a space where students and clients feel comfortable exploring and can find a pathway into the body they inhabit and the impact it has on the whole self.

References

Ferreira J.P., Ghiarone T, Junior C.R.C., Furtado G.E., *et al*. (2019). Effects of physical exercise on the stereotyped behavior of children with autism spectrum disorders. Medicina (Kaunas), 55(10), 685.

Girdler S.J., Confino J.E., & Woesner M.E. (2019). Exercise as a treatment for schizophrenia: A review. Psychopharmacology Bulletin, 49(1), 56-69.

Mehren A., Reichert M., Coghill D., Muller H.H., Braun N., & Philipen A. (2020). Physical exercise in attention deficit hyperactivity disorder: Evidence and implication for the treatment of borderline personality disorder. Borderline Personality Disorder and Emotion Dysregulation, 7, 1.

Subject Index

Note: illustrations are referenced by page numbers in *italics*

Author Index